KRAVTSOVA ANTONINA

Technologies
of Salvation and
Harmonious Development

Derivative work on materials
of the Teachings of Grigori Grabovoi

2017

Kravtsova A.I.
"Technologies of Salvation and Harmonious Development". Derivative work on materials of the Teachings of Grigori Grabovoi. – 2017 – 95 p.

Awareness of any actions immediately attracts man to understanding of his involvement into salvation of the world through the technologies of macro salvation, which Grabovoi G.P. gives. Derivative work was written on materials of the Teachings of Grigori Grabovoi "On salvation and harmonious development". Lectures read by Grigori Petrovich Grabovoi in 2002 are used as a basis:

April 16, 2002: **"Lecture 1. Introduction –** for lecturers of initial training".

April 23, 2002: **"LIT. Lecture 2.** System of salvation and harmonious development of Grigori Grabovoi. Methods of control by means of concentration on numbers or creation of number series".

May 14, 2002: **"LIT. Lecture 3.** System of salvation and harmonious development. Control by means of phrases. Eight methods".

May 22, 2002: **"LIT. Lecture 4.** System of salvation and harmonious development. Technology and methods of control by means of color".

May 27, 2002: **"LIT. Lecture 5.** Technology of salvation and harmonious development. Methods of control by means of sound and forms".

Salvation technologies of Grigori Grabovoi are given for understanding of very simple truths that are available to everyone. On the basis of recommendations given in these materials, methods and technologies of the Teachings can be easily and widely transferred to other people for understanding of the ways to recover health and normalize own events, and any events, at the level of macro salvation.

Jelezky publishing UG, Hamburg

www.jelezky-publishing.com

1. Edition, september 2017. - 56 p. © 2017, Jelezky publishing UG (Publisher), Hamburg

2017-1, 28.09.2017

ISBN: 978-3-945549-44-5

CONTENT

Introduction

Grabovoi Grigori Petrovich, the author of the Teachings "On Salvation and Harmonious Development" was born on November 14, 1963 in Kirovsky settlement (Bogara village) of Kirovsky district, Chimkentsky region, Kazakh SSR.

Grabovoi Grigori Petrovich is the Doctor of Physics and Mathematics, academician, author of discovery of creating sphere of information and original works on forecasting of futurities, their control and correction.

Grabovoi G.P. is the exclusive owner of registered trademarks «GRABOVOI®» and «GRIGORI GRABOVOI®» within the territories of the European Union, Japan, China, Australia, the USA (http://goo.gl/S2oKnz).

G.P. Grabovoi's recorded results on accurate extrasensory diagnostics and preventive forecasting, control over the events by means of generation of bio-signal and thought emission are given in the first three volumes of the book "The Practice of Control. The Way of Salvation". Recorded results of the practitioners of the Teachings of Grigori Grabovoi are given in books "The Practice of Control. The Way of Salvation", volumes 4, 5, 6 (http://goo.gl/aLSJSu).

The Teachings of Grigori Grabovoi "On Salvation and Eternal Harmonious Development" was written *"especially for everyone to have a chance to save himself and to be provided with the technologies of eternal development; and he/she must act as the Creator acts, because it is the system which shows the way of eternal development».*

Method 49 of G.P. Grabovoi's work "The Methods of Promotion of Grigori Grabovoi's Works in Social Networks" (http://goo.gl/SClPq1) shows that for promotion of the Teachings it is possible to promote one work, and then all the rest. Of course, there are works which are advisable to start learning the Teachings of Grigori Grabovoi with, for example – already mentioned "The Practice of Control. The Way of Salvation", "Unified System of Knowledge" – http://goo.gl/GN40bu, "Applied Structures of the Creating Field of Information" – http://goo.gl/V5qfsp, "The

Resurrection of People and Eternal Life from Now On Is Our Reality!" (https://goo.gl/MkTdJN)

Man may become interested in any work of Grigori Petrovich – as far as people have different levels of training, different interests: maybe someone will want to create Eternity at once on the basis of paintings from Grabovoi G.P.'s albums "Manifestations of Eternity" – http://goo.gl/yNKnoI, and someone is interested in work "Living Cosmosociology of Spiritual Creativity of Russia" http://goo.gl/1E5cfI and so on.

The choice of a certain work for promotion, for example, in Facebook may be done on the basis of the scheme given below.

The course of lectures for lecturers of initial training is of interest

Method 49 of G.P. Grabovoi's work "The Methods of Promotion of Grigori Grabovoi's Works in Social Networks"

The education sphere

The information from souls of all people

The Promotion of Grigori Grabovoi's Works

318549219714 9

Method 49 of G.P. Grabovoi's work "The Methods of Promotion of Grigori Grabovoi's Works in Social Networks" shows that for promotion of the Teachings it is possible to promote one work, and then all the rest.
The choice of a certain work for promotion, for example, in Facebook may be done on the number series – 318549219714 9

because salvation technologies for understanding of very simple truths that are available to everyone are given in it. Control takes place at the expense of formation of structure of own Consciousness.

The Author of the Teachings shows in his lectures the technologies with the use of control systems, such as concentration on numbers, work with letters, phrases, words, control systems with the use of colors, sounds and forms. The technologies in derivative work will be shown as they were given by the Author, because the sequence in understanding is very important. Studying the material and understanding it, man learns to see the schemes of control over spiritual vision or simply understands that he/she already possesses spiritual vision for a long time.

The fact is that during control, as Grigori Grabovoi says, *"mechanisms broadly known from each man's birth are used, i.e. mechanisms of thinking, and they are, generally speaking, exist as though automatically".*

The course of lectures analyses control system and in fact organization of such form of collective reality, which exists eternally, it means that each man must live eternally in his physical body. So all technologies of the course of lectures are aimed at prevention of probable global catastrophe. This created level means that the value of physical body should be made something like priceless and unavailable for destruction. This is the level of offered education.

2. Main phases of control

There may be such a variant of logically simple scheme that future processes are shown in the form of numbers: for example, two plus two is four. Four is an action that some would think is distributed into the future. That is, we are doing the following now: we are counting "two plus two", but receiving "four" in future. This example forms many associations. It means it is possible to make control on a finite object of action.

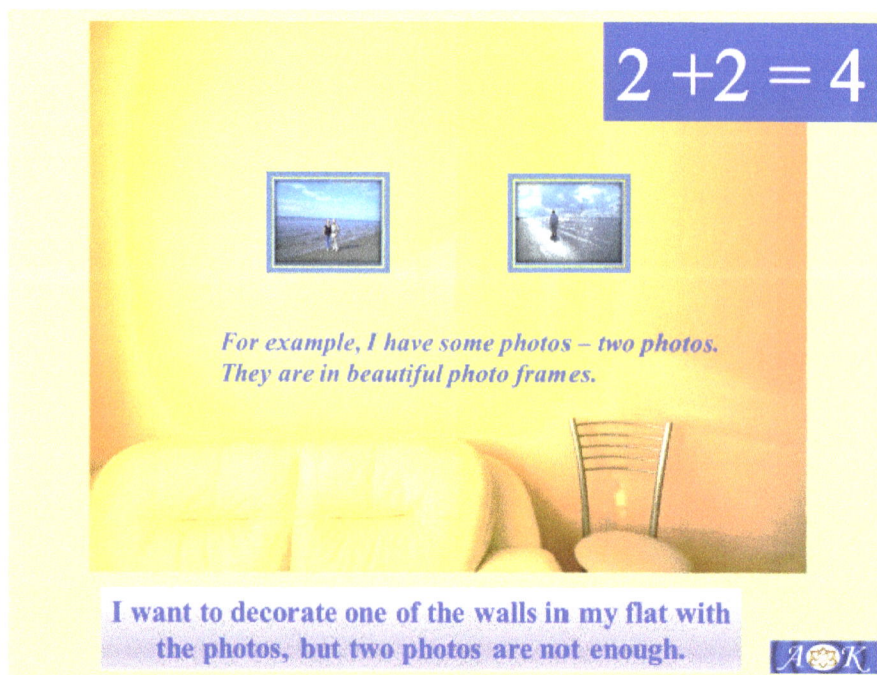

2 + 2 = 4

For example, I have some photos – two photos. They are in beautiful photo frames.

I want to decorate one of the walls in my flat with the photos, but two photos are not enough.

For example, I have some photos – two photos. They are in beautiful photo frames. I want to decorate one of the walls in my flat with the photos, but two photos are not enough. I concentrate on number "four" to receive a harmonious decoration of the wall. What do I need for it? First of all, the world must exist, it means that there is a house where I live and there is a decorated wall in this house.

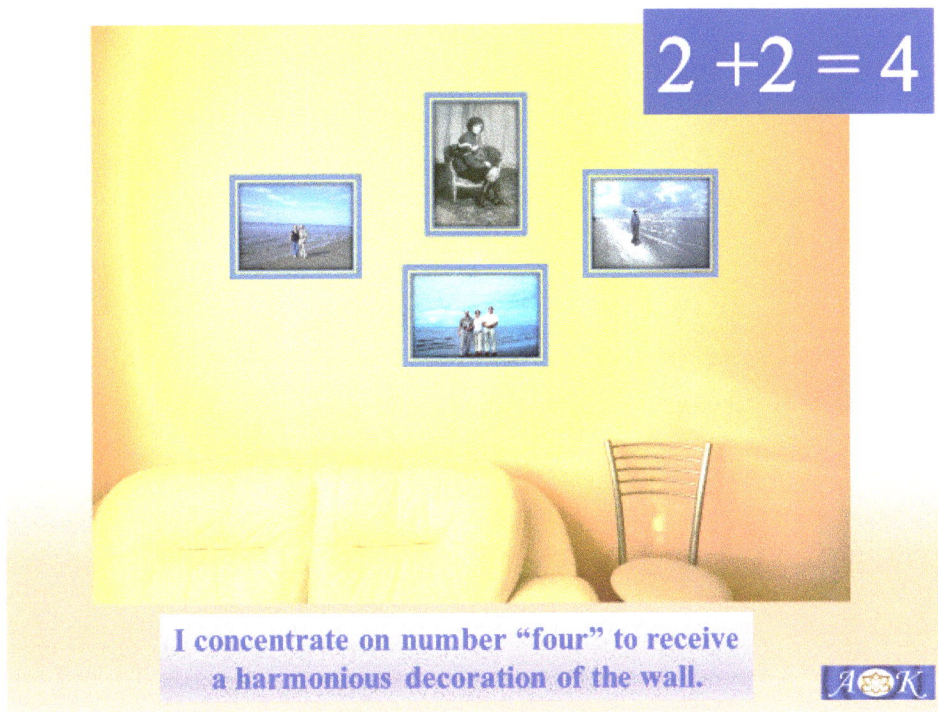

$$2 + 2 = 4$$

I concentrate on number "four" to receive a harmonious decoration of the wall.

It turns out that in number "two" I insert macro salvation for house simply to be on the planet, I concentrate on "four" – it is a solution of my task, my project. And I need to do solution: I decorate two more photos into frames that are in harmony with existing ones. "Plus two" is the way, the action which must be made.

Of course, there are people who will say – why so difficult? In truth man thinks over everything that was made by logics, and way without control becomes longer, because level of task realization is not laid down clearly. During practice of control the task is solved as if by itself: photos and frames are chosen – in my example – necessary accessories are bought in the necessary shop. And now the task is solved.

This simple arithmetic operation may be applied, for example, to understanding of technology of salvation, having laid down understanding into "four" and associated action of addition with inclusion of new technologies.

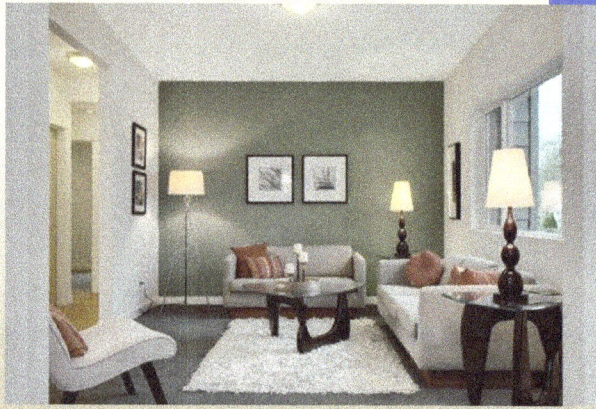

2 + 2 = 4

2 macro salvation

+ 2 The way to a solution of my task

4 The solution of my task

The concentration on a finite action.

"Plus two" is the way, the action which must be made.

The simplest first technology is the control with concentration on a finite object of action. And the example: man goes to the shop to buy a necessary thing. Stages of actions may be designated by spheres. Naturally, according to the system of macro salvation the first sphere is the sphere of macro salvation and eternal harmonious development for the house to exist simply and for us to develop in this house harmoniously. That is, man creates for himself such a level of work, such a flow of Light.

The second sphere: man must go out and pass the way to the necessary shop. And, finally, a certain, tenth or in our example third sphere, third number – he buys necessary thing in the shop. It is enough to concentrate on number "three", while understanding where to go and what to do: then man receives control.

Awareness of any actions immediately attracts man to understanding of his involvement into salvation of the world through

Stages of control for buying a necessary thing

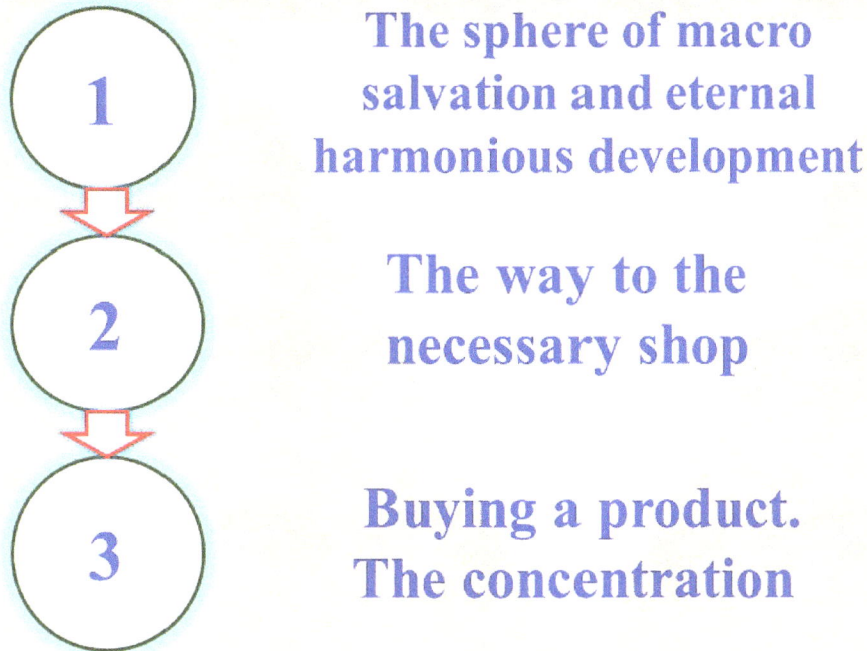

1 — The sphere of macro salvation and eternal harmonious development

2 — The way to the necessary shop

3 — Buying a product. The concentration

A K

the technologies of macro salvation, which Grabovoi G.P. gives. And it is clear for man that this very projection of future in logical perception gives control. We can see on the scheme given that the Light of macro salvation is the level of control.

"And then everyone will, first of all, understand very simple logical reason in the structure of your Consciousness: that if everything exists that was made by the Creator, then it is the very way which is simply like an open door which already exists – people already live at the level created by the Creator. This means only development and action in direction of the Creator's goal, and the goal of the Creator is eternal life and eternal development of everyone".

A special attention in the first lecture is paid to the fact that provision of the future interval of development is a necessary element of control and any form of reality possesses such element as **necessary element of own existence.** Salvation from probable global catastrophe is the minimum necessary control element, because if global catastrophe takes place, then the whole planet can be destroyed.

Consequently we really talk about salvation of the world, but not of a single planet. So, after completing this task first, then private control systems are realized, where solution of situation exists – simply control to achieve private control task exists.

3. Control over event system at the level of macro regulation. Notion of level of number "eight"

Even implicitly man may solve the problem set, improve health and receive direct help by understanding the tasks of macro salvation.

Notion of level of number "eight"

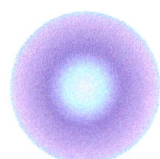
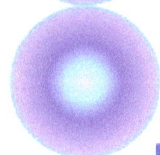
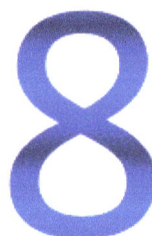

Upper part is an organization of something like an eternal control level

Lower part of "eight' is a level of private tasks

For example, you have a certain task – to receive knowledge, know how to process knowledge, and then transfer to eternal distribution – this is upper part of number "eight".

To carry out control privately – for example, there can be private events – there is lower part of number "eight".

"Structure of time is the system included in the event information." To receive a possibility to control immediately by salvation tasks, one, first of all, should set his mind to the fact that such possibility exists, and, secondly, such possibility is necessary for the systems of quick or immediate transfer of knowledge.

The idea of eternal development is a state of Spirit which can provide for such development of the state of Soul and the state of

Consciousness, which can technologically create reality, regulate any situation around you, both external and internal, and self-organize, for example, physical body.

There is a notion of "eight" level, and there is just a number "eight", that is, upper part is an organization of something like an eternal control level, and lower part of "eight' is a level of private

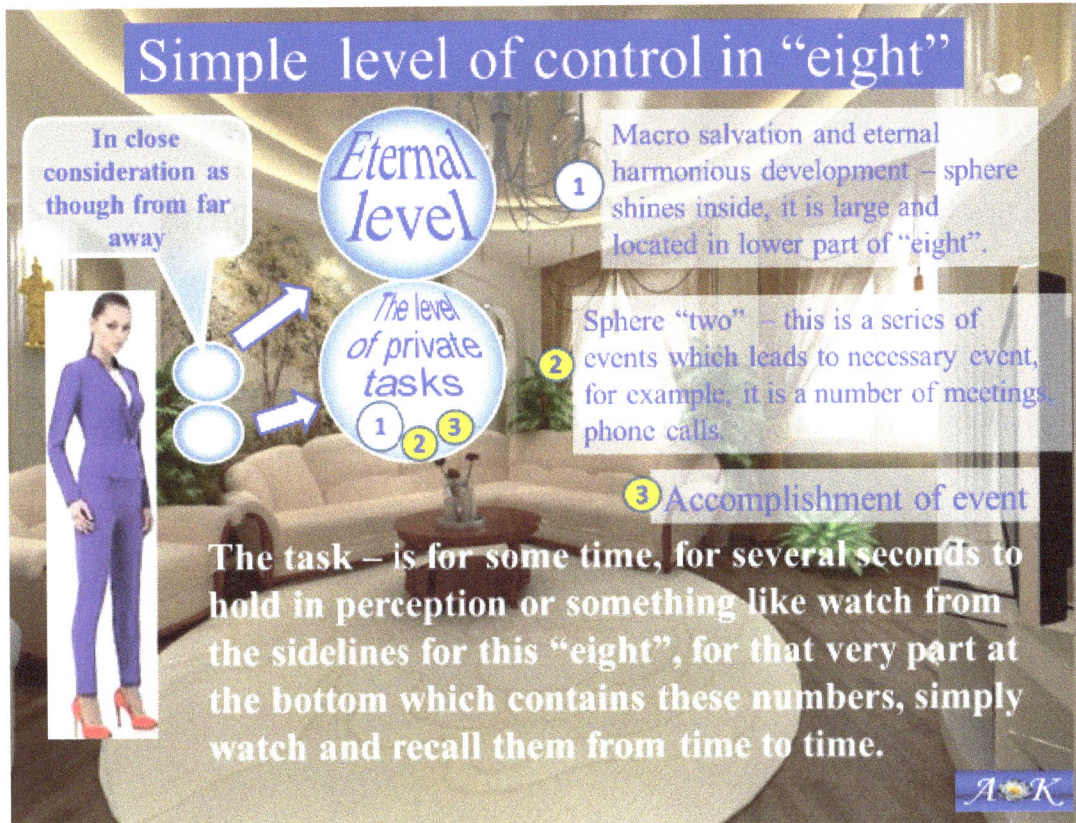

Simple level of control in "eight"

tasks. For example, you have a certain task – to receive knowledge, know how to process knowledge, and then transfer to eternal distribution – this is upper part of number "eight". To carry out control privately – for example, there can be private events – there is lower part of number "eight".

Man just has number "eight" in his thoughts or his perception. Control lies in fact that there is lower part of number "eight" for private events. In close consideration as though from far away one may see principal items of events.

In lower part of number 'eight' which is usually located vertically, we fasten our eyes on, as though imagine the events that we want to receive. On the scheme "eight" is located in front of physical body of man – opposite to heart. So, we distinguish principal items of events in lower part of "eight".

1 – macro regulation: sphere shines inside, it is large and located on the left. Two other spheres are smaller.

2 – this is a series of events which leads to necessary event, for

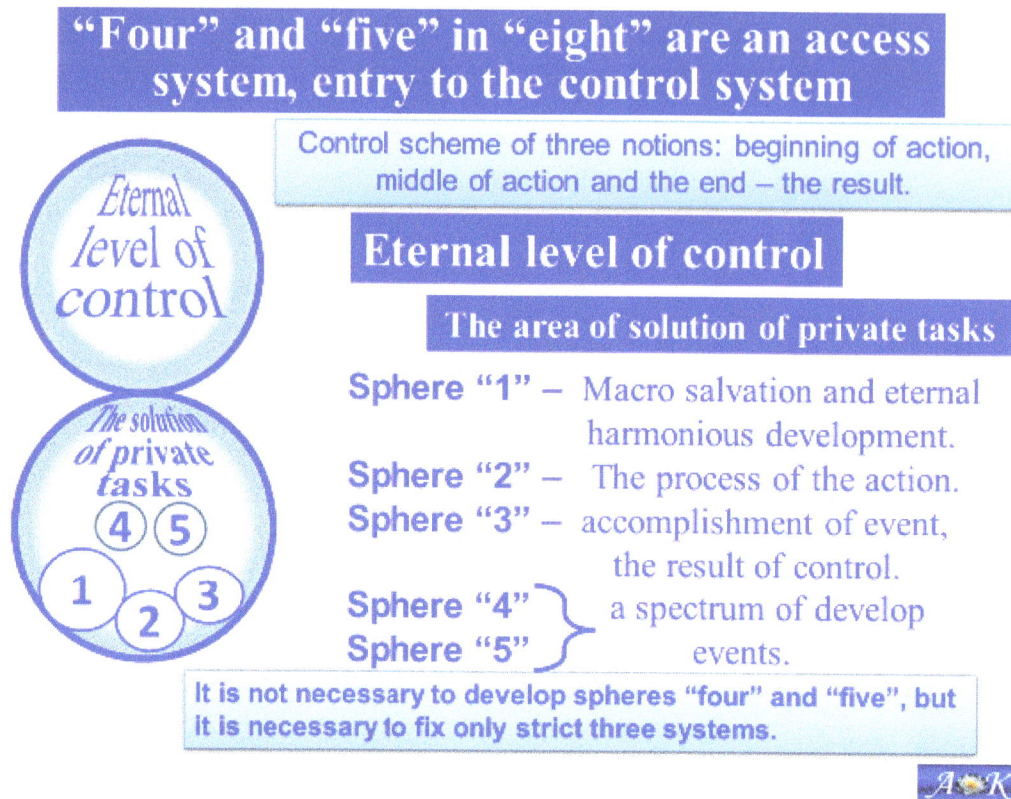

"Four" and "five" in "eight" are an access system, entry to the control system

Control scheme of three notions: beginning of action, middle of action and the end – the result.

Eternal level of control

The area of solution of private tasks

Sphere "1" – Macro salvation and eternal harmonious development.
Sphere "2" – The process of the action.
Sphere "3" – accomplishment of event, the result of control.
Sphere "4" ⎫ a spectrum of develop
Sphere "5" ⎭ events.

It is not necessary to develop spheres "four" and "five", but it is necessary to fix only strict three systems.

example, it is a number of meetings. The second event may include several meetings, that is, a certain number of events, meetings, calls that must be performed from the point of view of man who makes control. Man determines himself when it should happen, but anyway, it is better to work with a number of events at certain time. It turns out that time is included into accomplishment of events in sphere "two".

3 - accomplishment of event.

The task of the man who makes control after assignment of events is for some time, for several seconds to hold in perception or something like watch from the sidelines for this "eight", for that very part at the bottom which contains these numbers, simply watch and recall them from time to time.

An example concerning certain event is given in the seminar: it is necessary to do so that certain information which will be able to save really, including from local catastrophes, was received by EMERCOM of Russia. So, we fix "eight" at the certain level of perception near physical body, highlight lower circle and three spheres in the circle, that are presented on the scheme and are described earlier: macro regulation, the second one – sphere of EMERCOM, and the third one – number "three" – certain technologies arrive to EMERCOM and they use them.

It is possible to add two actions in control – "four" and "five" – just in case so that to take into account positions which develop from optical form of information. We perceive the object optically, not by means of sounds, we definitely imagine: we see in perception. We fix for several seconds one sphere – it is the first, then two – the second sphere, then the third one. Just in case we fix two numbers on the top – "four" and "five' that mean something like a spectrum of events.

Any events can be placed into this scheme by reducing them up to three notions: beginning of action, middle of action and the end – the result. Added actions regarding development of events are also under control. In this technique the main spectrum of control is added – how to get into control system? The element is in that numbers "four" and "five" are added, that is, what develops. It is not necessary to be engaged in it, it is not necessary to develop it, but it is necessary to fix only strict three systems.

The system is perceived easily in terms of understanding: you can move this number "eight" in perception near physical body and find the point of the highest activation, for example, near the heart, at the distance of 20 cm from physical body.

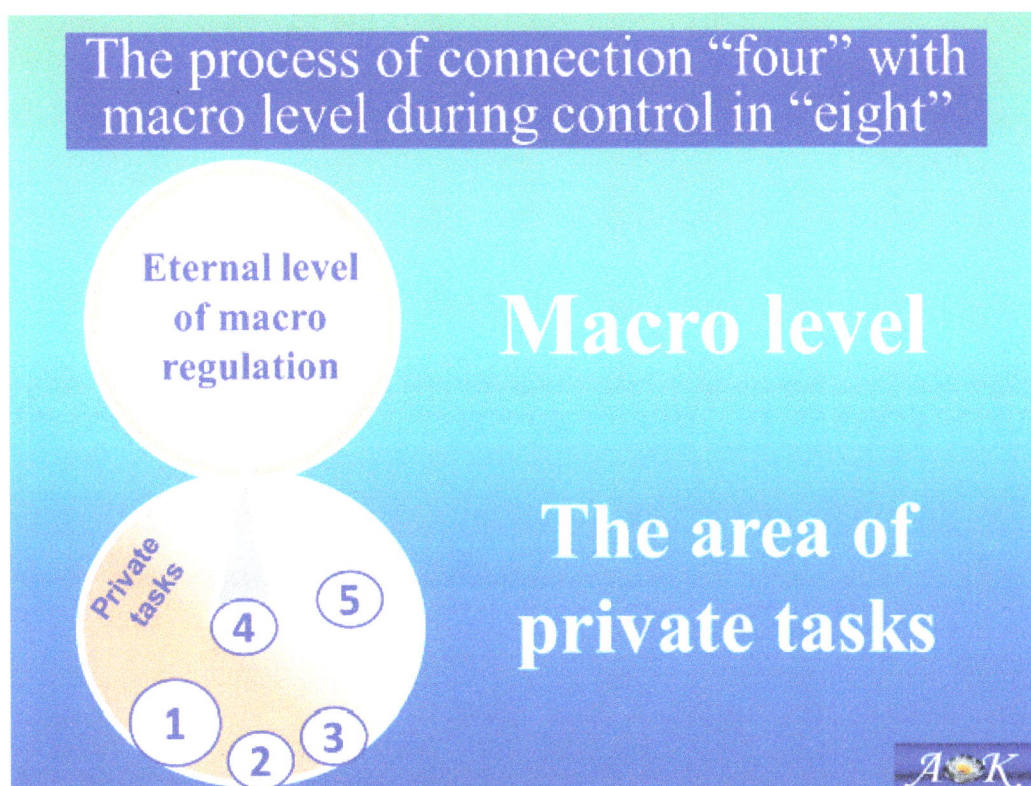

The process of connection "four" with macro level during control in "eight"

Eternal level of macro regulation

Macro level

Private tasks

The area of private tasks

4 5
1 2 3

A K

Hold "eight" and go along all the numbers once again. Situation control is that the numbers "1", "2", "3" and "eight" are fixed, and

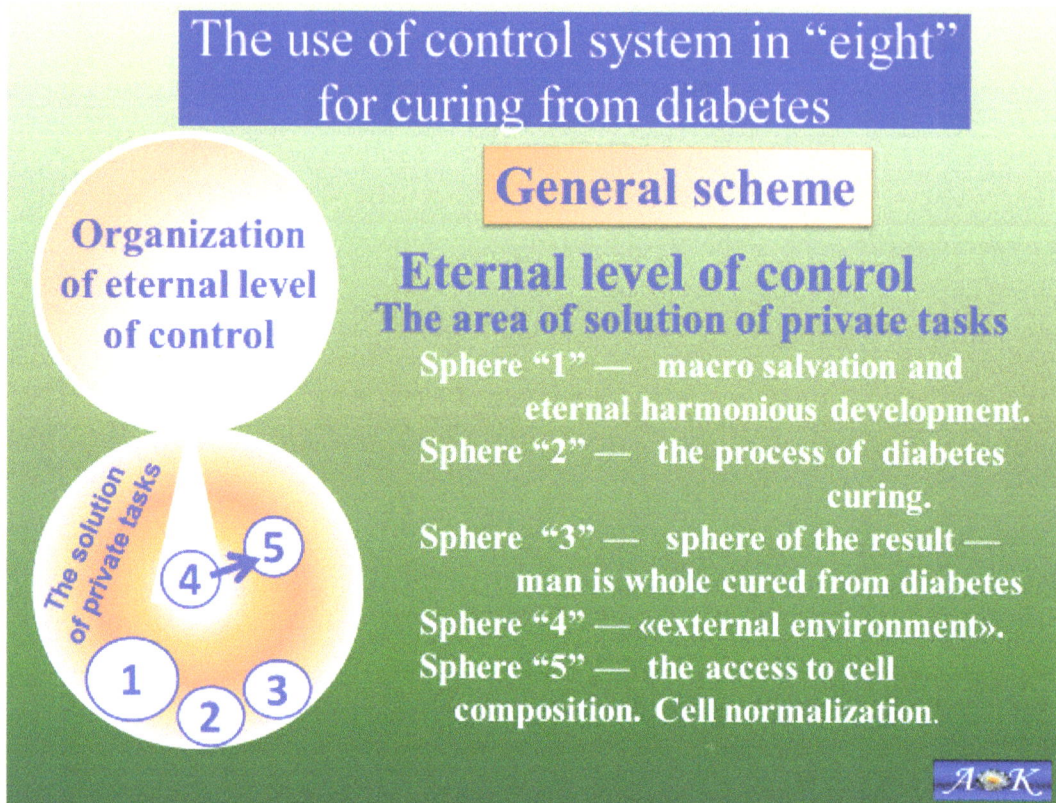

The use of control system in "eight" for curing from diabetes

General scheme

Organization of eternal level of control

The solution of private tasks

Eternal level of control
The area of solution of private tasks
Sphere "1" —   macro salvation and eternal harmonious development.
Sphere "2" —   the process of diabetes curing.
Sphere "3" —   sphere of the result — man is whole cured from diabetes
Sphere "4" — «external environment».
Sphere "5" —   the access to cell composition. Cell normalization.

"four" and "five" can be moved. Control is performed by simple moving of "four" inside the circle. At that moment, the moment of "four" moving, one may see the light coming from the level of macro sphere. Man starts practicing and seeing how the process of connection with macro level is developed, how the result is developed and so on.

Let's analyze an example from the seminar: the use of control system for curing from diabetes. To carry out control actions let's immediately make "eight" and three numbers in lower part in our perception. It doesn't have to be diabetes, you make take another disease.

Control scheme for diabetes curing: macro sphere is the number "one". Macro regulation sphere is the level which does not change. "Two" is the task to treat diabetes, "three" – man is cured. "Four" and "five" are an access system. It is possible to get to man's events through "four", so, "four" is his event surrounding. "Five" is a cell composition.

Work, that is, look through only "four" and "five". Concentrate your attention on "four" – cell composition opens up: *"and it is immediately clear what shall be regulated, for example, in cell composition. Let's say, simply the amount of liquid phase shall be regulated in any specific cell. It is not necessarily to look into morphology of cell. It is clear that there is more liquid there than necessary. You simply perceive it as information, it is the system of access to information."*

Of course, the author's text of G.P. Grabovoi should be studies, then additional or precise understanding through the words, through the sound opens up. What is desirable to understand here? Two slides show the Light approaching to the sphere, which is designated as "external environment". Moving "four" in lower part of "eight", we find that position of it, which develops the process of connection with macro level, that is, with upper part of "eight". As far as we need to go to cell level, then (it would be clear later in the text) we go to the level of general connections with collective reality. It was explained a little bit earlier than current control concerning treatment of diabetes.

Once again - "four" and "five" are an access system. After working with "four" we rise to cell level. As far as *"the system of access to information"* is in "five", then we'll work in "five". That is, we need, let's say *"to regulate the amount of liquid phase in any specific cell"* or simply normalize the cell to the standard of health, if we work with another diagnosis.

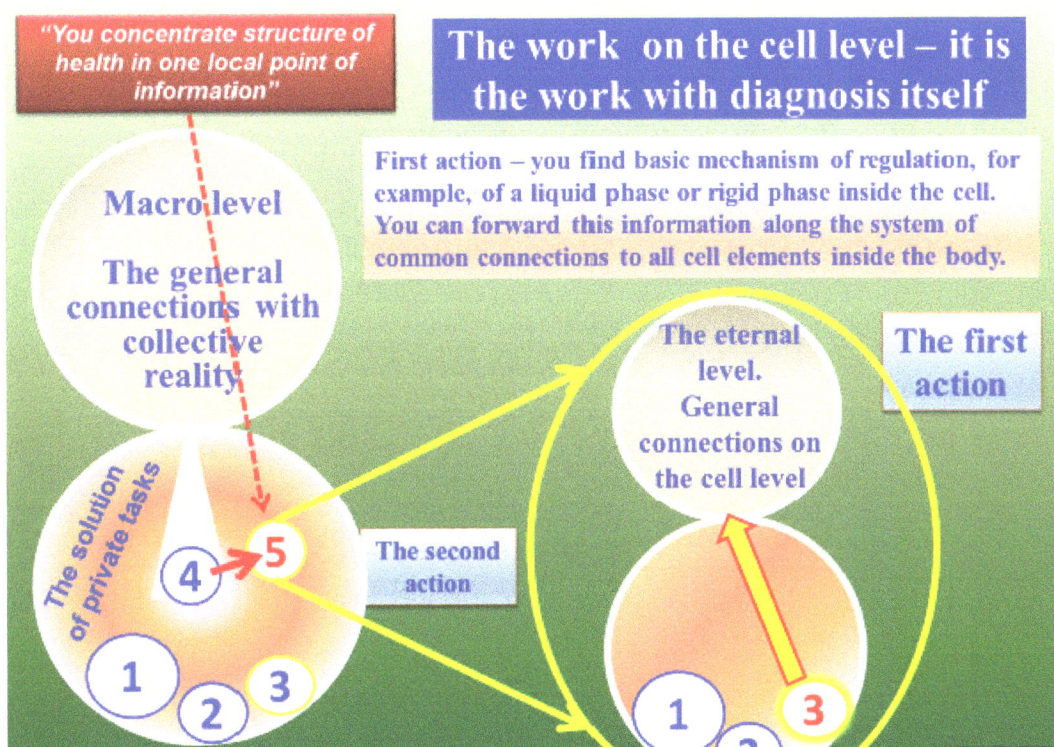

"You concentrate structure of health in one local point of information"

The work on the cell level – it is the work with diagnosis itself

First action – you find basic mechanism of regulation, for example, of a liquid phase or rigid phase inside the cell. You can forward this information along the system of common connections to all cell elements inside the body.

Macro level

The general connections with collective reality

The solution of private tasks

The eternal level. General connections on the cell level

The first action

The second action

17

And then it is said in the seminar: *"when you need to regulate, you again go back to "eight" already in that level".* On what *"that level"*? On the one that we together came to through the access system: that is in level of "five", if it is possible to call it so, in fact we went to the level of access to information. And then, precisely according to the author's text, as far as every word there gives not only control preciseness, but preciseness of information transfer is observed:

"We again have sphere "one", it is left number "one"; put the task of regulation in "two", that is, normalization of liquid phase of cell, from which diabetes is cured; and the third one is once again the same, yes?... health man. And it turns out that you concentrate structure of health in one local point of information. From the point of view of common connections you really mend collective reality so that man becomes healthy. It is as if the second action in control".

I think that local point of information will be that very sphere "five" where we made the second control action. Here we shall understand the connections and the levels of control, because we went to collective reality through the Light to "four": on the same level we worked in "five". So, after our control on cell normalization the light according to the law of universal connections went into collective reality – there where eternal level of control is organized.

"And the first action is that you really control at the expense of the fact that as soon as you find basic mechanism of regulation, for example, of a liquid phase, or let's say, rigid phase inside the cell, you can forward this information along the system of common connections to all cell elements inside the body.

It turns out that you work in this case not even with certain cell, but simply work with diagnosis itself. And when you make such an action, stability appears, that is sphere of recovery – the third point – it simply starts shining. That is, you can see that you made necessary action at the given period of time. Number "three" becomes shining – the number itself, it simply becomes apparent immediately. So, you made a control in respect of, for example, treatment of diabetes".

Actions and the sequence of these actions are clear from the control scheme. Main regulation mechanism is offered us by Grigori Petrovich Grabovoi in his seminar. Through the access system –

numbers 4 and 5 – we entered regulation level: but at first the access system was built. And the first control action takes place right on the cell level in "five". Here man immediately learns spiritual viewing, spiritual vision and understanding that in any space, for example, in small sphere one may make control which leads to curing. Control takes place in information space of "five".

Understanding of the author's text may be different from the offered one, any additions may arise, but, of course, the original should be thoroughly studied. This work represents one of the variants of control understanding.

4. Creation of sequence of numbers for work with any situation

Sequence of numbers for work can be created on the basis of control method in "eight". Information is universal in terms of understanding. *"And the system of concentration on numbers, for example, "Human organism recovery by concentration on numbers", is that very universal system of normalization which spreads irrespective of man's characteristics, that is, irrespective of age, situation or event construction".* If some people have a diagnosis – it is possible to exclude the structure of diagnosis from the general level of Collective Consciousness with the help of sequences of numbers consisting of seven digits.

It is offered to see individually how numbers are connected, where in series of numbers, for example, in seven-digit system, macro regulation sphere is located: sphere "one" may be found there, sphere "two" – where it is located, and so on.

Creation of sequence of numbers for work with any situation may be started with the studying of method of work in "eight": there are 5 numbers inside it: 1, 2, 3, 4, 5 – and together with "eight" there will be six numbers. *"And we must introduce one more number, where is 'eight" located, on what is it located in Consciousness?"* In Consciousness "eight" always goes after "seven", so, we add 7, that is, we receive seven-digit number series.

"If we want to add to this system something like two degrees of freedom and make strengthening in action, that is, in development, we may find the eighth number, which is in truth "eight" itself, or

add "nine", which is the development of this "eight". And we can create number series with the help of very simple method, simply by denoting the carrying platform – this number "seven".

Then the control is performed, a mechanism of series obtaining is performed. What kind of mechanism is it?

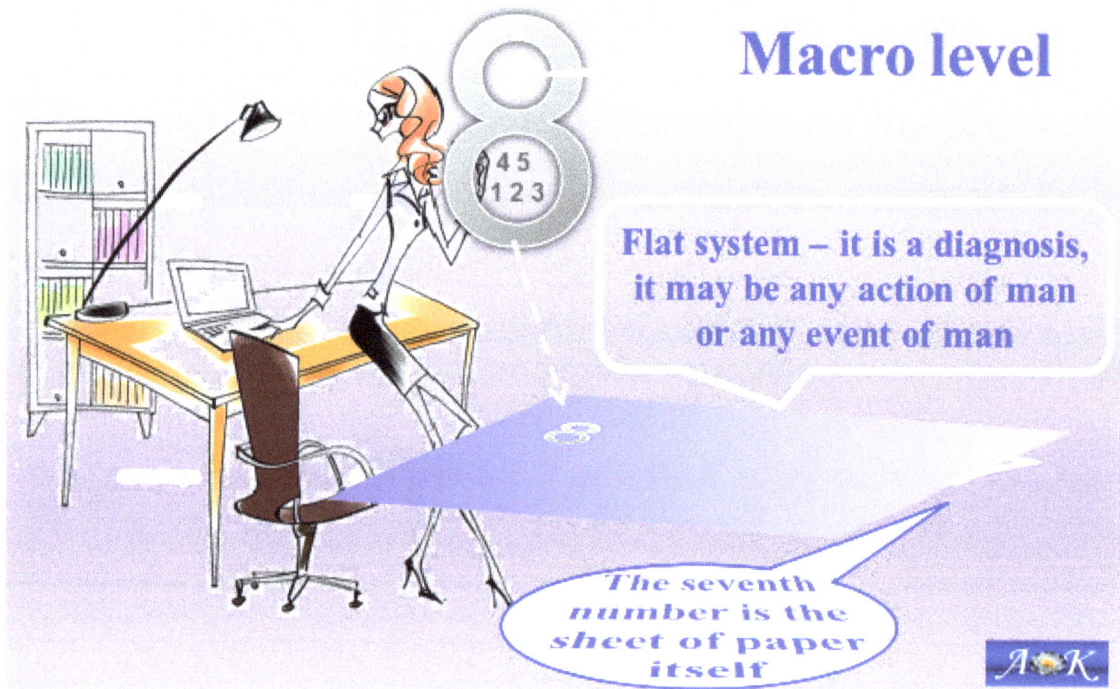

Creation of sequence of numbers for work with any situation

Macro level

Flat system – it is a diagnosis, it may be any action of man or any event of man

The seventh number is the sheet of paper itself

We need to receive a projection series. We take "eight' with numbers inside it - 1, 2, 3, 4, 5 – and shake in hand for a long time: figuratively. We remember from the previous technology that "eight" possesses an eternal level with all connections we need right in this work and "eight" also possesses the level of solution of private task. In upper part of "eight" we placed the level of macro regulation.

When we shake "eight" with numbers, we remember what is placed in it, and then we simply throw numbers on a flat sheet and watch how they are placed. *"It is something like a mechanism of this shaking, mechanism of throwing, it is always one and the same for a certain diagnosis, because we throw on a sheet of a certain diagnosis. And while they are falling they very strictly and certainly arrange in a certain horizontal variant".*

Flat sheet is not necessarily a diagnosis, it may be any certain action of man: to go somewhere, do something, organize something and so on. With such a very simple method we may throw numbers on horizontal system and use these numbers as controlling ones.

Event for control is placed in front of you and it is better for such event to be represented in the form of sphere for the beginning. You took an event in sphere from the table, for example, and turned into a plane, into a sheet. *"Every man knows what event he wants to emphasize".* You emphasized event, then took this event as a sheet of paper. There is "eight" and five numbers in it, the seventh number is the sheet of paper itself. We must throw numbers on this sheet of paper. *"In principle, numbers something like place themselves according to a certain law... in respect of one and the same event".*

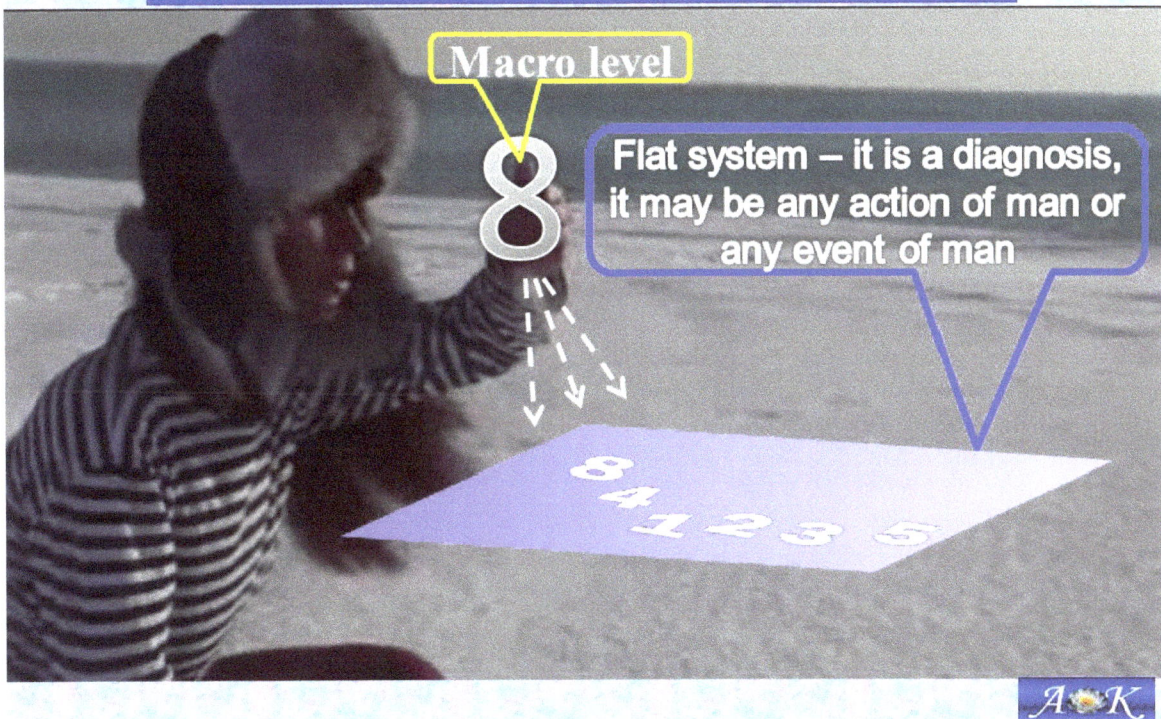

Creation of sequence of numbers for work with any situation

Macro level

Flat system – it is a diagnosis, it may be any action of man or any event of man

We take any one number, for example, "eight", and throw it on the sheet for several times: the number falls on one and the same local place, that is, is does not fall at random. As soon as "eight" is placed, we start throwing the other numbers one by one – and several throws determine the sequence of numbers.

Any number can fall on one and the other place – this is a variant of event, so we should increase control over the event. There can be strict numbers, but there can be those that move. We need to fix the system and work in this system of numbers. By the way, it is possible to work with "eight" in three-dimensional system in spatial connections or in two-dimensional one, but in perception, that is, not to put it on plane.

5. Work with letters to receive a desired event

Number is stricter in perception, while letters start something like moving, so it is more difficult to hold phrase in visual perception, you should make certain efforts.

The system existing in perception for work through the words and the system for work on plane – they are close in terms of the technology of use: there is no need to activate anything in terms of access to physical space. After formulating any control goal rather clearly it is possible to keep it in perception, or it can be written down. As soon as we write down or keep the phrase in memory, then control lies in concentration in upper part of letters at the level of macro regulation: the letters are conditionally divided by a line along the axis of symmetry into upper and lower part. Concentration is made in lower part of letters successively on every two letters.

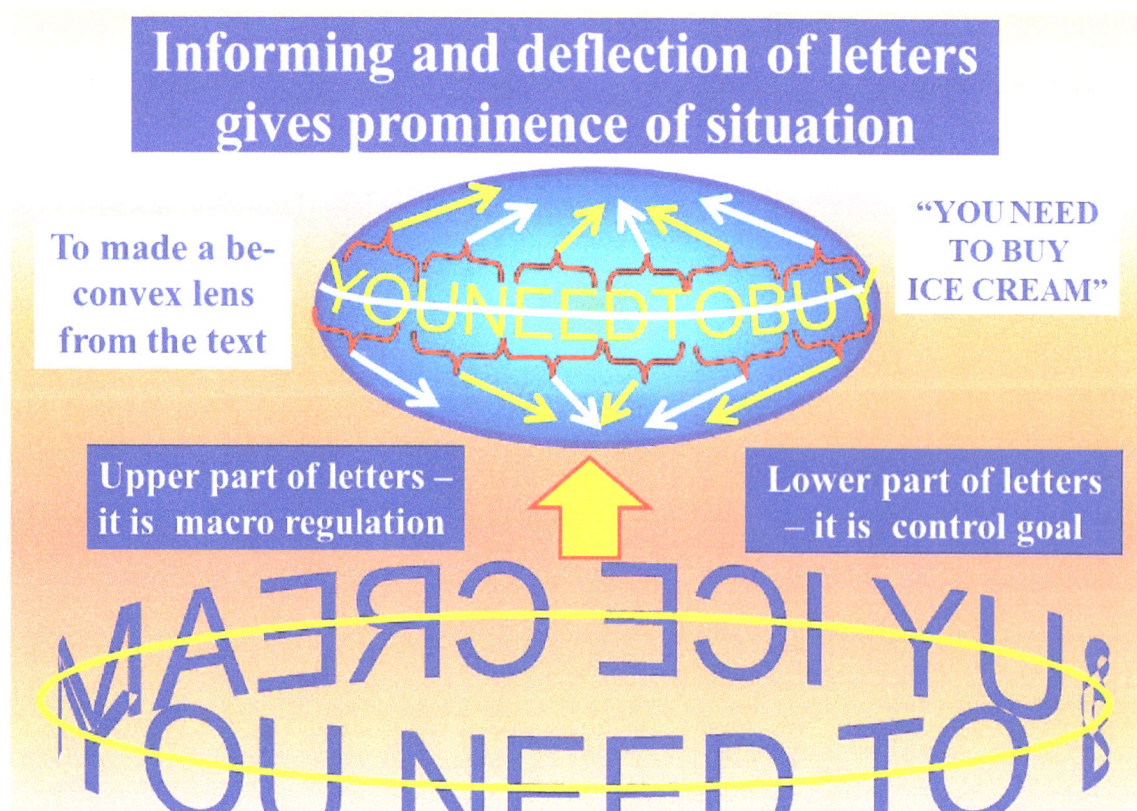

Informing and deflection of letters gives prominence of situation

To made a be-convex lens from the text

"YOU NEED TO BUY ICE CREAM"

YOUNEEDTOBUY

Upper part of letters – it is macro regulation

Lower part of letters – it is control goal

"That is, for example Y, O – concentration takes place in lower part, that is, you as if pause your attention for a while, then leave, as if with the help of optic bean from Consciousness deflect, then make concentration for U, N… first of all illuminating upper part there – macro regulation, then lower part, then E, E; [D, T; O, B and so on]. And you as if deflected this word in such a way. That is in perception you have prominence as if from yourself. Unique lens in perception optics formed so as if you unbent perception boundary".

The boundary of perception is unbent, you receive greater deal of beams inside an actual system which arranges control goal. It is necessary to deflect all these letters in control phrase – and only by two letters. Make one step, then the other, the third one – until all these letters take the shape of sphere. It is necessary to catch the moment when the letters start taking the shape of sphere. *"As soon as this sphere is formed, it is necessary to control for it to go vertically up and at the level of your perception this sphere transforms into an*

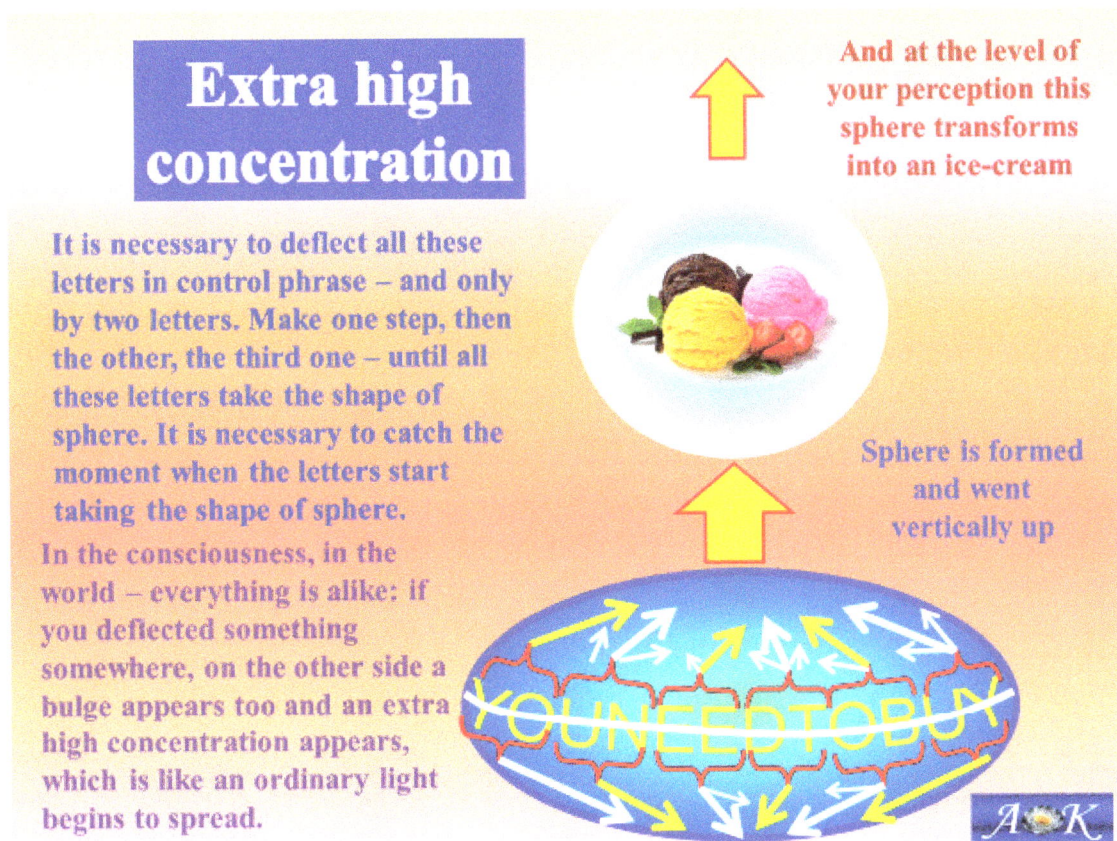

Extra high concentration

It is necessary to deflect all these letters in control phrase – and only by two letters. Make one step, then the other, the third one – until all these letters take the shape of sphere. It is necessary to catch the moment when the letters start taking the shape of sphere.

In the consciousness, in the world – everything is alike: if you deflected something somewhere, on the other side a bulge appears too and an extra high concentration appears, which is like an ordinary light begins to spread.

And at the level of your perception this sphere transforms into an ice-cream

Sphere is formed and went vertically up

ice-cream".

Salvation of everyone is the sense of upper part of letters, that is, control of event construction of macro regulation is just achieved by concentration on letters. Universality of this method and quick mastering of this system lie in the fact that just certain letters are used here.

Deflection of letters gives prominence of situation, just as well it is possible to work with the document, and with situation. For example, Grigori Petrovich gave a note to airport dispatcher with the request to postpone the flight of the passenger airplane on technical grounds. With the help of thought he made a be-convex lens from the text - by means of such deflection a note as if entered the dispatcher's information system the most prominently. The note was passed, dispatcher postponed the flight, though he was not to do it.

It means that it is possible to work through such systems in case of salvation of any situation – *"even the system which is not covered by the code of the organization works".* As soon as optics is developed – exit to control system – some external help arrives to prevent a problem in the form of supporting systems. The more man practices for the system of macro salvation, the more he improves his Spirit in terms of readiness to control the situation.

6. Color control

You must perceive color in case of color control. Color searching and perception of color are so that the principle is very simple and it looks like the principle of numbers sowing from the "eight". You take control goal in the form of silver sphere and appoint that control goal is inside of this sphere. Sphere can be in any universe, at the level of man's perception, but it would be better to locate near physical body.

When you formed control goal, you start sowing, that is, we must percept color of control goal. Color can be not the only one in perception: first of all it can be light purple, then green, then any shades can be. During letters control the method "by two" was used, that is, we deflected by two letters. And here - the first, the second color appeared, they must be fixed. After fixing the first two colors we as if cut the others, *"we didn't allow development of such scenery in our Consciousness ... - like in a movie – we turned off the player".*

And this is the control by goal: first of all you make silver white color in goal, then leave this sphere in front of you and wait till the first and the second colors appear, that will be able to expand infinitely. Remember the first two colors, sort out all the rest, and transfer two colors to the Spirit. The Spirit remembers and knows that there were two colors.

Then control takes place through these two first colors and it is realized. You don't have to do anything further, because color in

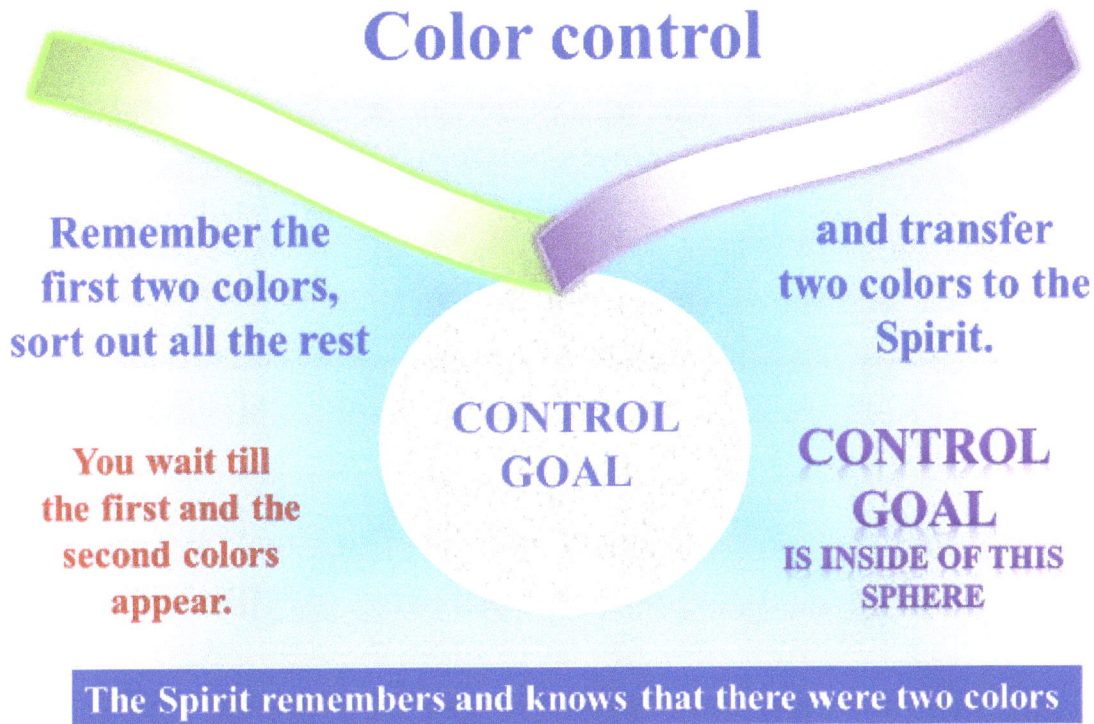

Color control

Remember the first two colors, sort out all the rest

and transfer two colors to the Spirit.

You wait till the first and the second colors appear.

CONTROL
GOAL

CONTROL GOAL
IS INSIDE OF THIS SPHERE

The Spirit remembers and knows that there were two colors

man's perception possesses a feature of infinity: color has no size and it is the closest to spiritual perception of information.

And principle – why two? – because it is the principle from the Creator. When we talk about the second – it is all the development of the World. So we work just as the Creator works: "one – two". There are two letters, there are two colors there – and this is the principle of Creator's work. *"And why particularly the second is really the whole technology? To create just one microelement, it is necessary to know the whole technology of the World, right?... the development of the World. So in this case we work exactly by two elements"*.

7. Work through sounds and forms

"Work through sounds and forms includes some kind of generalization and commonality". Working with forms, for example, with number, letter, color, man works at the level without organization of any perceived system, so there is a maximum simplicity in mastering, in access, because there is no need to fix them somehow. On the other side, there where the system is not formed, one should have an extra high concentration of Consciousness in terms of logics of actions, task of actions.

The principle of work with sound lies in the fact that pre-sound system is determined first: one simply takes and makes control goal so that this goal gets into system which exists before the sound. And what forms the sound? For example, one may strike a cord, turn on sound-reproducing equipment and form sound, but these are the elements of physical world, manifested one.

The situation of control over elements of reality as if physically exists, because Grigori Grabovoi gives control over all elements of reality. In sound control we approach the problem that this is something like a control over the result, that is, element-sound, which should be at first created – find a guitar with at least one string or turn on the sound in any equipment. Here we can see a very simple law of matter creation, creation of reality by the level as the Creator makes it.

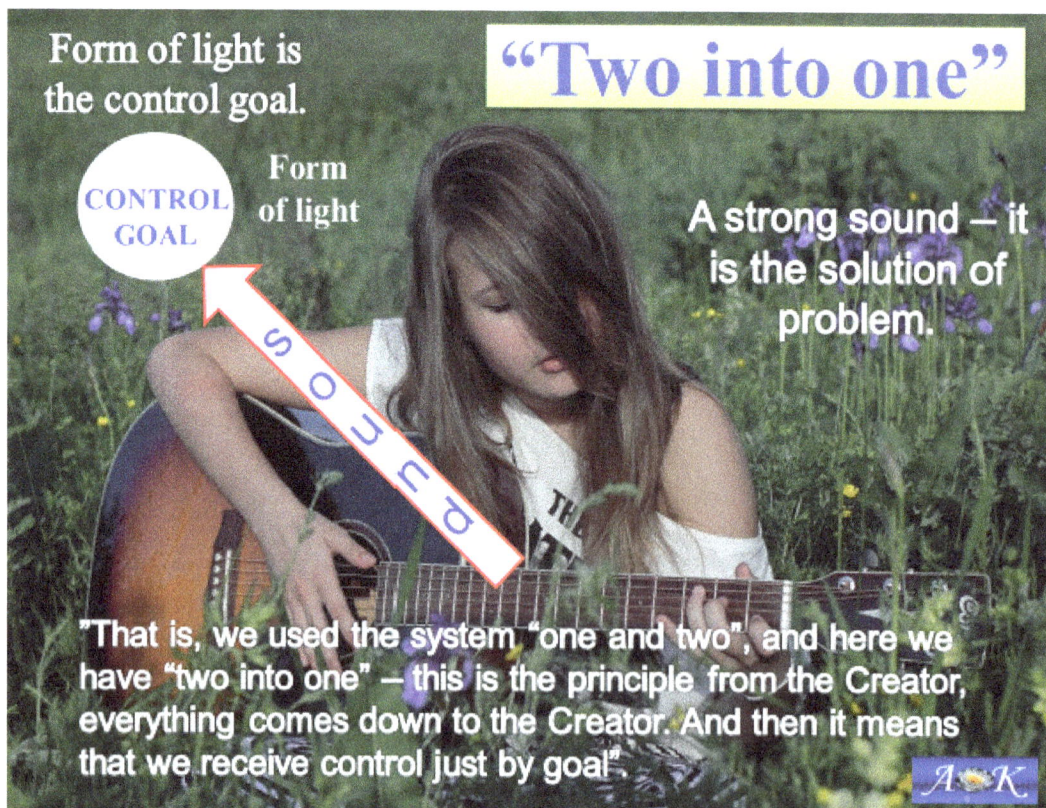

Form of light is the control goal.

CONTROL GOAL

Form of light

sound

"Two into one"

A strong sound – it is the solution of problem.

"That is, we used the system "one and two", and here we have "two into one" – this is the principle from the Creator, everything comes down to the Creator. And then it means that we receive control just by goal".

A K

To create reality one should have that structure, that state of Spirit, such state of Soul, that is, have the Soul which was created by the Creator. Sound is formed from something. If we can perceive color as the color of sky, then sound in perception of man is the element also created. And so we arrive to the fact that creation of sound is the sound form, *"that is, we can create sound by a form in our perception.*

And when we take the form of Light, simply highlight the form of Light and create the sound, then at the expense of form movement we may, generally speaking, create melody, and this melody is something like control. Well, you may create not only melody, you may create a sound, for example, a strong sound – it is the solution of your problem, where form is the control goal. And combination of form and sound – you have combination of "two into one", right?.. that is, the other way round. That is, we used the system "one and two", and here we have "two into one" – this is the principle from the Creator, everything comes down to the Creator. And then it means that we receive control just by goal".

Let's take any task of our own. We perceive intensity of sound and see the form of this sound. Regulating the form, we change intensity. We are as if in the wave of concentrated control. In our mind we may catch the sound, which corresponds to the solution of the task set, while we move the form which corresponds to control goal, it is simply any form.

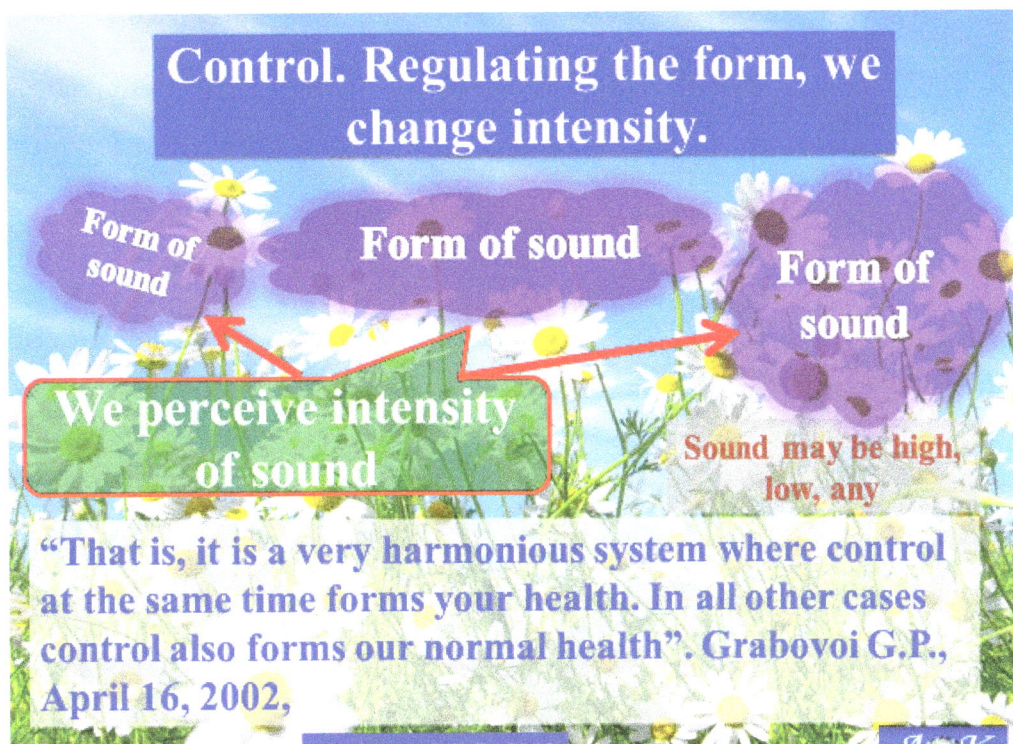

Control. Regulating the form, we change intensity.

Form of sound

Form of sound

Form of sound

We perceive intensity of sound

Sound may be high, low, any

"That is, it is a very harmonious system where control at the same time forms your health. In all other cases control also forms our normal health". Grabovoi G.P., April 16, 2002,

27

Sound may be high, low, any, but it is better for sound to be multidimensional. It is not necessarily a certain melody, though it is possible to transform sound in a famous melody, which we remember at spiritual level, but you are not obliged to remember, you may simply transform into a famous melody and fix it. Sound is tuned simply by motion of form – just as the guitar or any instrument is tuned up. Tuning the sound up we see and understand that this control really takes place with this sound.

Sound control has a long-lasting effect. You can simply see sound in perception. Sound perception is perceived by a certain ear close to physical body and it is formed so that just as according to the law from the Creator the element of reality forms the very body of man. *"That is, it is a very harmonious system where control at the same time forms your health. In all other cases control also forms our normal health"*.

Man listens to sound by a physical body, external sound is at the same time an internal sound. *"It turns out that external one creates internal reality, that is, man's body. In such a way you can see how transition into the structure of eternal development takes place, where the principle of development is laid down in the very eternal development that each action is so that it is directed into eternity because it is infinitely. And at the same time it forms a local system – both You, that is, man and your external appearance, level: for example, the world, people, social standing and so on"*.

It is advisable at once to practice control which affects macro interests, that is, the principle of macro salvation must be realized. This information is given in details at the Author's seminar of G.P. Grabovoi dated April 16, 2002: **"Lecture 1. Introduction.** – for lecturers of initial training".

METHODS OF CONTROL BY MEANS OF CONCENTRATION ON NUMBERS OR CREATION OF NUMBER SERIES

8. Methods of control by means of concentration on numbers

The first level of creation of number series structure is the following level: how the Creator acts. So, it is necessary to create fundamentally a number series which is in principle simple for its control and ensures availability of many factors of control. According to the law of connection of any information with all external and internal information of area: the more general influence man exerts on the system, than the more precisely, quickly and correctly in terms of time he receives the result of control.

The principle of action of number: the first parameter – the number itself contains macro control information. The second parameter – any sequence of numbers is saturated with macro control information, it is as if highlighted in Consciousness or the man who makes control concentrates more on it.

As for private tasks, everything is exactly the same. Concentration on numbers is a private task: healing, control over events, it can also be any macro control task, I mean subtask, something like subarea, can be the whole macro control area too.

If we analyze a simple operation of addition: to receive number "nine" we need to add five to four in logical perception. *"Then, in principle, if nine is the area of macro control for a certain period of time, then we can consider that for an autonomous system, for example, five is also an area of macro control, if we do not perform an operation of addition".*

Here we pay attention to the fact that macro area is a resulting area too. When fundamental principle of number organization is taken into account, then maximum number of systems is covered, and a very simple system which takes into account all parameters acts as a support.

Control task is an infinite transfer of accurate information too. Number system allows doing it correctly. And educational level, the level of knowledge transfer is laid into the system of macro control. It is always desirable to organize universalism in spiritual perception of the method and each method may be realized in any case.

Grigori Petrovich Grabovoi offers his methods from his practice described in the work "The Practice of Control. The Way of Salvation".

9. Creation of number series

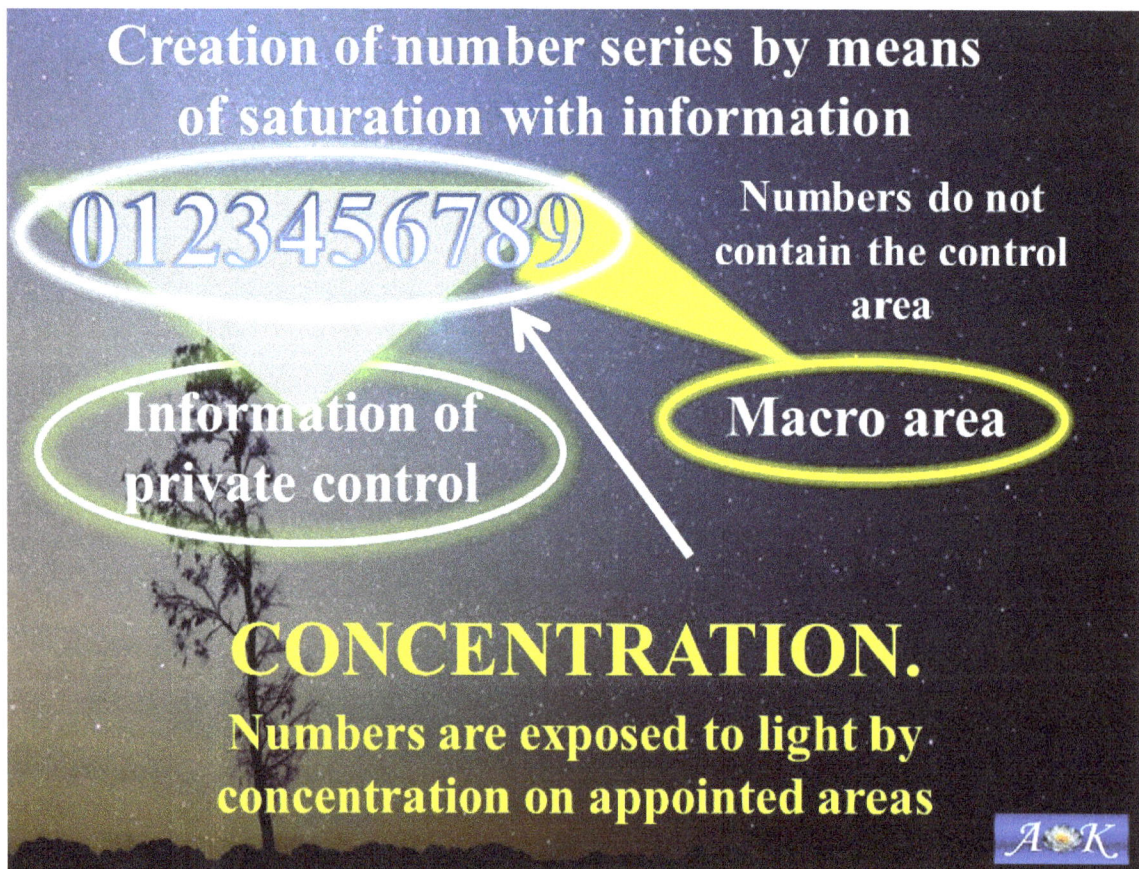

Creation of number series by means of saturation with information

0123456789

Numbers do not contain the control area

Information of private control

Macro area

CONCENTRATION.

Numbers are exposed to light by concentration on appointed areas

"The method lies in the fact that you create a number series by means of saturation with area of macro control. That is, numbers in

this case do not contain macro area, and you simply create a number series and saturate, for example, macro areas, certain numbers with information, and it means that you saturate some other numbers with private information, private control. That is, in this case numbers do not contain the very control area".

The first action is the creation of number series. The second action – numbers are saturated with area of macro control and the area of private tasks is created. The next action – numbers are exposed to light by concentration on appointed areas. You can imagine or write down the numbers on paper and work with paper.

9.a. Fundamental principle of series creation

Let's analyze the principle of number organization: there is an initial point of organization of any reality. This initial point possesses an absolute value.

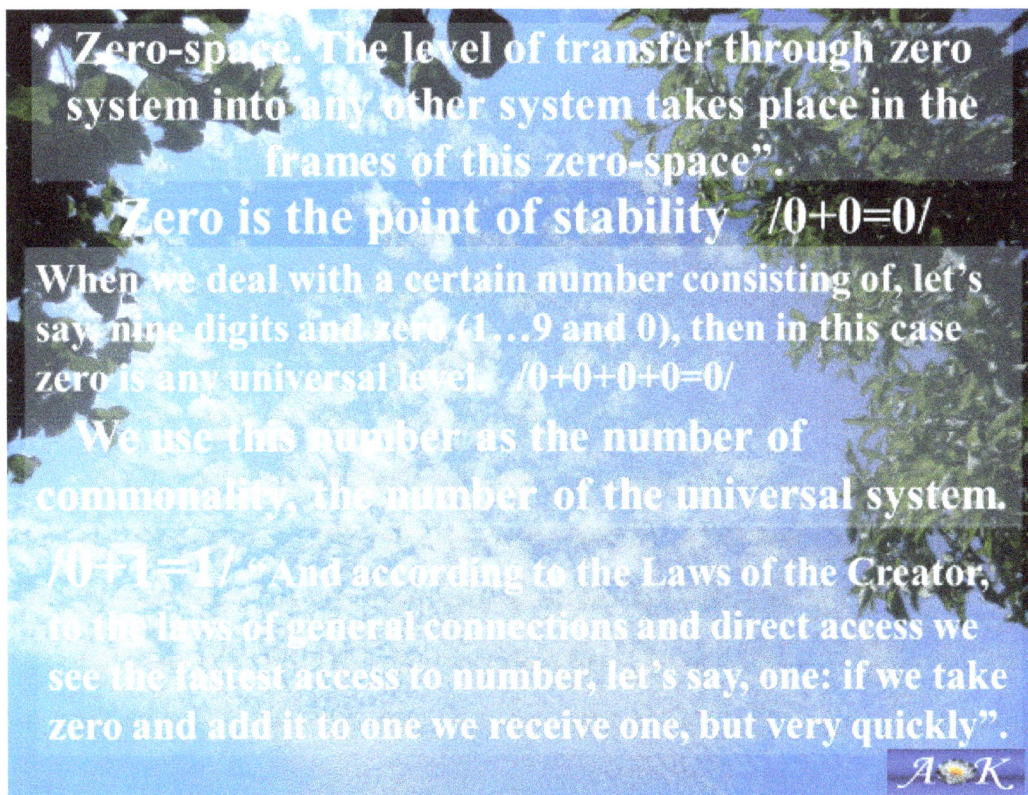

Zero-space. The level of transfer through zero system into any other system takes place in the frames of this zero-space".
Zero is the point of stability /0+0=0/
When we deal with a certain number consisting of, let's say nine digits and zero (1...9 and 0), then in this case zero is any universal level. /0+0+0+0=0/
We use this number as the number of commonality, the number of the universal system.
/0+1=1/ "And according to the Laws of the Creator, to the laws of general connections and direct access we see the fastest access to number, let's say, one: if we take zero and add it to one we receive one, but very quickly".

"A notion of any universal level is introduced in this point. And this level should exist in a number or a number series".

"When we deal with a certain number consisting of, let's say, nine digits and zero, then in this case we deal exactly with the

principle of organization of such a universal space where rather universal properties from the point of view of number exist (in this case it is zero). That is, if we use this number as the number of commonality, the number of the universal system, then it is clear that if we, for example, add a great number of zeros, anyway we will receive zero, that is, some invariant space which does not change depending on external conditions. That is why in this zero space of thinking, let's call it zero space, the level of transfer through zero system into any other system takes place in the frames of this zero space".

The slide is offered not only to repeat or draw attention to information, but for a reader to understand that with own Consciousness it is possible to enter a zero space, just like, for example, the space of sky.

The texts of Grigori Petrovich are such that you simply want to repeat everything once again, without missing anything, but as far as we have the original, let's take only the key aspects so that to remember the meaning of given technology, and the reader will take all details, nuances and explanations from the original, from this bottomless fund of Knowledge. These methods are represented in the next Author's seminar dated April 23, 2002.

System controllability, namely access into any system in control will be obtained if any number will be placed near zero, and it can be placed from either side. Zero is the point of stability: zero plus one is one, and so on. There is a logic of control in Collective Consciousness that zero is a universal number which does not change the characteristics of adjacent number.

"So, we think that according to the laws of creation of absolute, I'd say, universal system, we can analyze zero number as such a system. And according to the Laws of the Creator, to the laws of general connections and direct access we see the fastest access to number, let's say, one: if we take zero and add it to one we receive one, but very quickly".

Characteristic of the next level of construction: number series must be located as systematic as possible and be more harmonious in respect to zero, and this is the principle of quickness in Consciousness.

10. Cross method

In this method, which is preliminary prepared, we build two number series, that is, we build systematically and harmoniously in respect of zero. In space of own thinking or simply on paper we place number series vertically and horizontally around zero, and put nine into the centre of zero (zero space) by conation.

We place numbers one, two, three, four from top downward to zero, and downward from zero – numbers five, six, seven, and eight. In the second series which is again crossed with zero, horizontally from left to right: one, two, three, four – these numbers up to zero, and numbers five, six, seven, and eight – to the right from zero.

"We made a crosswise construction, and it is zero that is placed inside. And then we start closing this system into control sphere. That is, in this case control sphere is such that, first of all, top and left parts of this crosswise location of number series are the control connected with macro regulation and right and bottom parts are the control of private tasks".

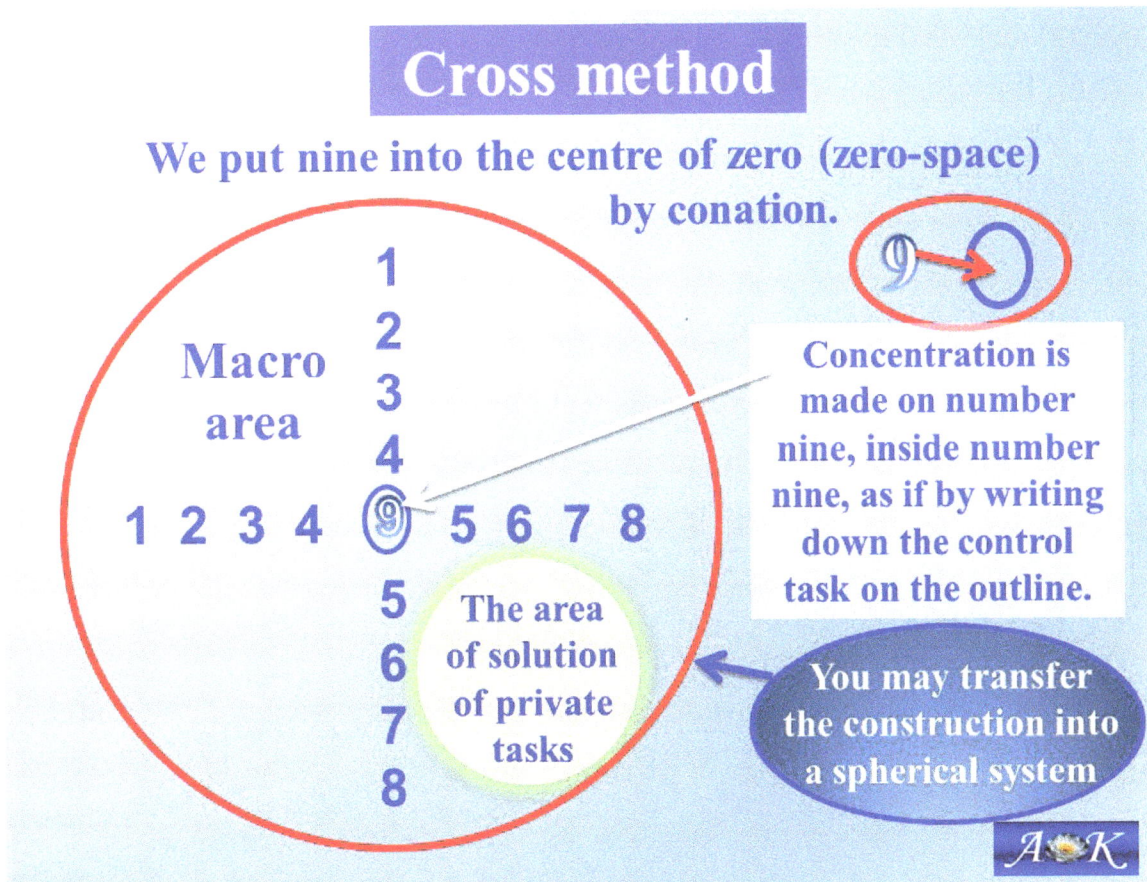

Cross method

We put nine into the centre of zero (zero-space) by conation.

Macro area

1 2 3 4

1 2 3 4 ⑨ 5 6 7 8

5 6 7 8

The area of solution of private tasks

Concentration is made on number nine, inside number nine, as if by writing down the control task on the outline.

You may transfer the construction into a spherical system

The slide given shows all construction of control system. The scheme is simple and clear. *"There is another sub-meaning of this control that there is control over private tasks in macro regulation, and visa versa – there is control over macro level in private tasks. In this case it is carried out through number nine, which is located inside zero. So, you tied the system, more simply, you created a node in control information which means a stable and continuous action, because through number nine you made a peculiar kind of bunch of control elements, and such one which permanently saturates control goal".*

Numbers five, six, seven, and eight are included into the level of private task solution, so some subtasks can be specified on these numbers, and the goal itself, as it was told earlier, is written along the outline of number nine. Saturation of right lower level can be done spiritually, you can write a control scheme especially for yourself. Concentration is made on number nine, inside number nine, as if by writing down the control task on the outline. And this action takes place inside zero.

We received a stable control system. What does it mean? We have a set goal, a set task, but there is an event series to solve this task. In case of overlapping of this system on the event series the most principle systems in events are revealed. That is, man easily chooses important events from many events leading to solution of control goal and denotes them with numbers five, six, seven, and eight.

"Thus according to the laws of the Creator you create practically eternal construction. Eternal construction means its universalism and repetitiveness as well as stability during the processes of eternal development. So, this construction works exactly on the basis of these conditions".

So not to control the whole control system you may transfer the construction into a spherical system, but do it so that to make immediately eight and place this construction into its lower part. You received control through number eight.

G.P. Grabovoi shows in his seminar control practice according to protocol No. 07/92, page 41, volume 1, three-volume edition "The Practice of Control. The Way of Salvation". Based on the protocol an airplane was diagnosed by side number so that to detect any defect and the rate of the airplane over certain period of macro control system in whole. Macro control system is the whole information

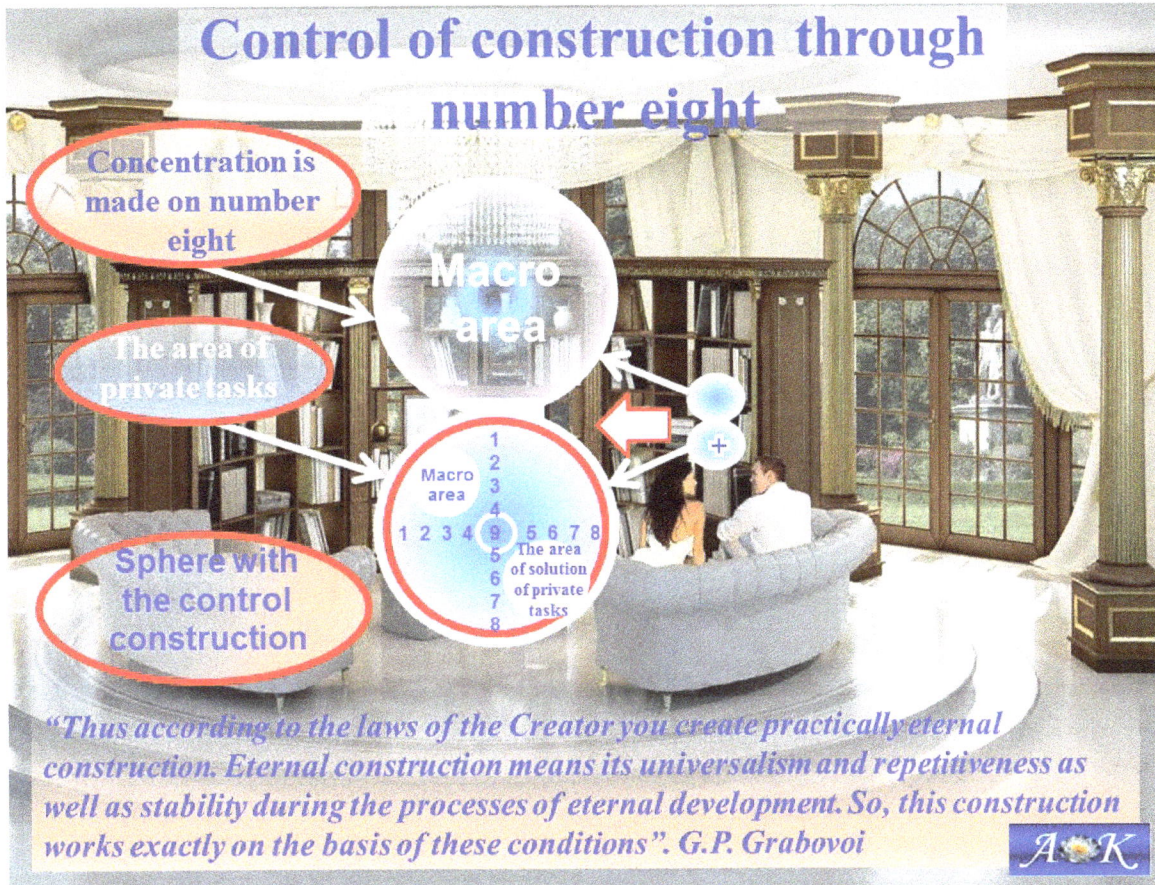

Control of construction through number eight

Concentration is made on number eight

The area of private tasks

Sphere with the control construction

Macro area

Macro area

1 2 3 4 5 6 7 8

1 2 3 4 5 6 7 8

The area of solution of private tasks

"*Thus according to the laws of the Creator you create practically eternal construction. Eternal construction means its universalism and repetitiveness as well as stability during the processes of eternal development. So, this construction works exactly on the basis of these conditions*". G.P. Grabovoi

where probable global catastrophe is absent.

Controlling over safety of flight we shall connect number one in the side number with number one in macro area. Control takes into account just the spatiality of perception, that is, number series is viewed as the whole series. The side number is crystallized in this number system on the left and top, just like according to the system of special crystallization the level of optical perception is distributed. The control scheme represents the result of introduction of the side number into the control system. It is important to understand that the whole information is introduced into the area where probable global catastrophe is absent.

Horizontal part of the series to the right from zero corresponds to the level of the main systems, and numbers five, six, seven, and eight of the vertical series correspond to the level of private, certain problems connected with airplane units themselves.

"Simply it is necessary to determine, at the very least roughly, what corresponds to any number in the airplane.

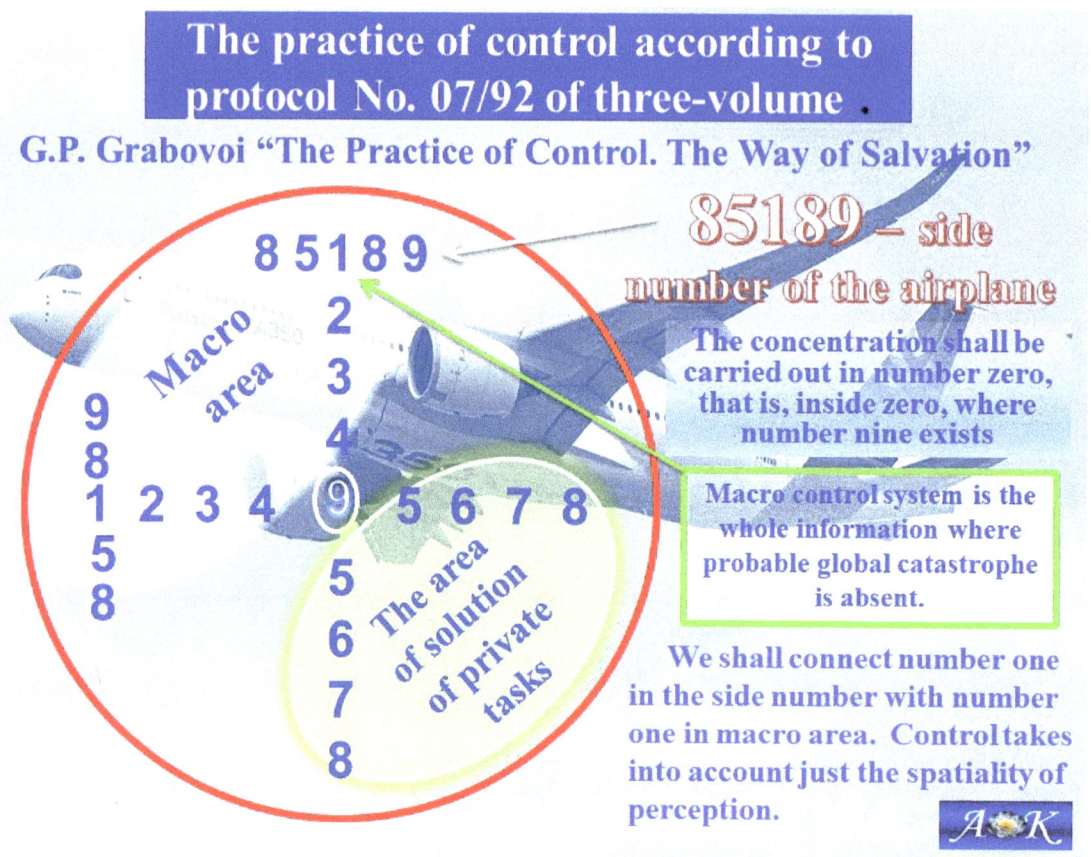

The practice of control according to protocol No. 07/92 of three-volume .

G.P. Grabovoi "The Practice of Control. The Way of Salvation"

8 5 1 8 9

85189 – side number of the airplane

The concentration shall be carried out in number zero, that is, inside zero, where number nine exists

Macro control system is the whole information where probable global catastrophe is absent.

We shall connect number one in the side number with number one in macro area. Control takes into account just the spatiality of perception.

And then you can see how control takes place. It is the control from the point of view of diagnostics and at the same time control for catastrophe not to happen. And here, for catastrophic level of information development not to happen the main concentration shall be carried out in number zero, that is, inside zero, where number nine exists, at first you make control that the plane does not get into catastrophe, then you make control moving along the number series from zero to the right or to the bottom".

In the same way you can carry out diagnostics of any machine, any event. You may write down the date of future events, for example the year, time and the date and test the number series from the point of view of what should be made a control element in the event. It is a general system not only for diagnostics but for creation of optimal factor of event series development, if you concentrate on nine.

11. Creation of trailing number series

Diagnostics can be carried out by means of creation of so called trailing number series. If we simplify the system by means of transferring on paper, anyway, we will receive comparable diagnostics, because we know what is going on there at the moment of such diagnostics.

Control diagnostics via trailing series looks so that from physical body of the one who makes control some paths start trailing in optically detected range. At first we set a control goal. The goal is to organize a number path for control goal: that is, a number path moving to event realization shall appear.

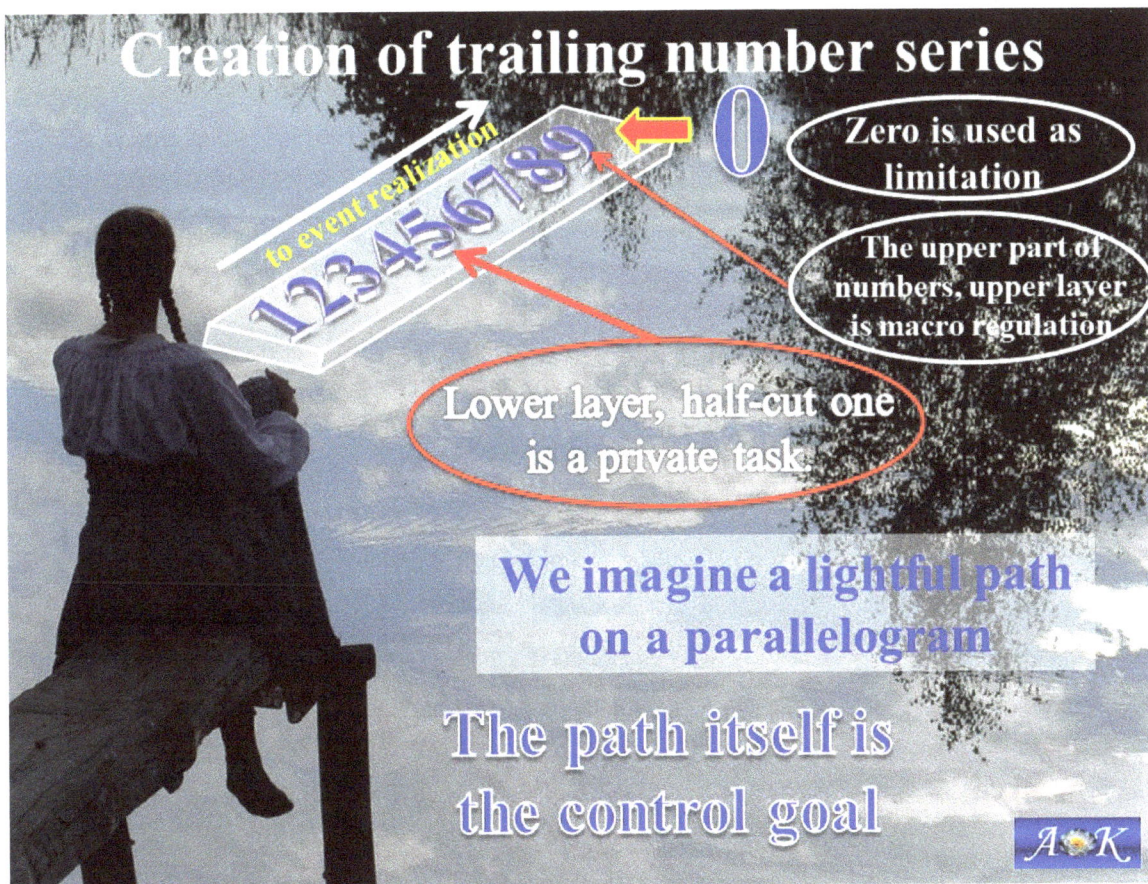

The principle of number series organization is simple: these are numbers from one to nine, and zero is used as limitation. Zero is at the end, and the series starts with one. The path itself is the control goal. We imagine a lightful path on a parallelogram which is rest on a highlighted optics. The upper part of numbers, upper layer is macro regulation, and lower layer, half-cut one is a private task.

So, as soon as we start placing numbers, then zero fixing at the end of our series starts acting so that a part of numbers starts as if relatively moving. We put numbers that start moving and build a number series for control goal located under this path. The principle is very simple: you should tune to your heart rhythm or to your arm movement, that is, you should tune to yourself.

As soon as you tuned to control goal and revealed it by the heart rhythm you can separate those numbers, which from one to nine are located on this path. Numbers shall be either raised or taken off this path and they shall be correctly placed. If event is close, then the principle of this control lies in the fact that you shall take the date of this event, and this event is separated from this composition of numbers: for example, using the date of month you take two numbers and move them into the base. It is the simplest and mechanized method comparable with notion of selection.

At the seminar the author gives the principle of diagnostics based on the scheme of a mine. *"And number series is a system which should show position of a number, position of number at given level and this number must mean something."*

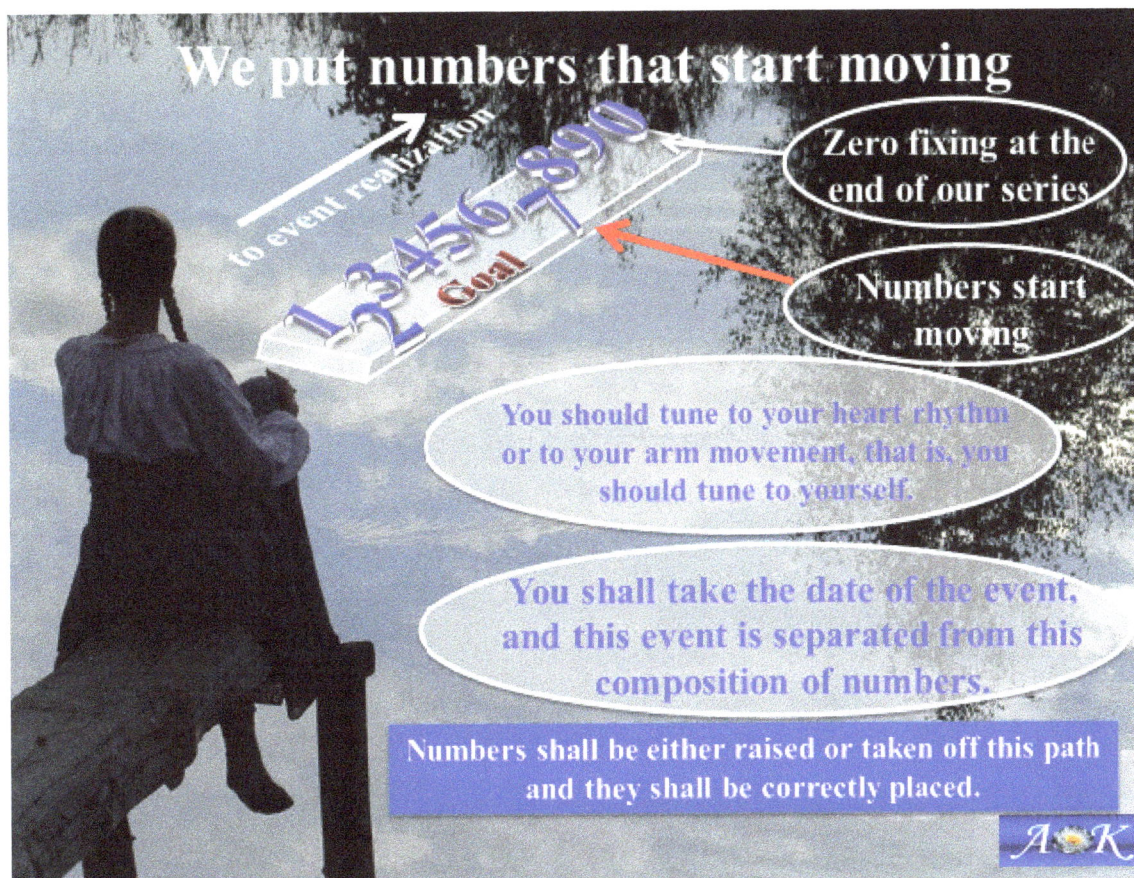

We put numbers that start moving

to event realization

1 2 3 4 5 6 7 8 9 0

Goal

Zero fixing at the end of our series

Numbers start moving

You should tune to your heart rhythm or to your arm movement, that is, you should tune to yourself.

You shall take the date of the event, and this event is separated from this composition of numbers.

Numbers shall be either raised or taken off this path and they shall be correctly placed.

Grigori Petrovich was given the scheme of the mine and asked to show the compartment where fire was and the compartment where people were. He put trailing series on the lightful path on the scheme of the mine, designated that number two will show the fire, and number one will show the compartment where people are. Numbers moved along the scheme and showed both compartments, people were saved.

Series must work on a base. In this case the mine scheme is the base. If man is in the mine he can, working with trailing number series, set the goal of finding a safe place where he will be saved from. The principle of work is represented on control scheme. For purpose of practicing on the basis of this technology man may find some information that is known to man beforehand.

The Author says the following about this method: *"in this case I showed the technology where a spiritual system works, that is, you work at the level of Spirit, Soul, Consciousness. And at the same time it's all about the fact that your body, I mean your system actualized in the form of physical body in case of action, reaction, development affects the system I have just told about".*

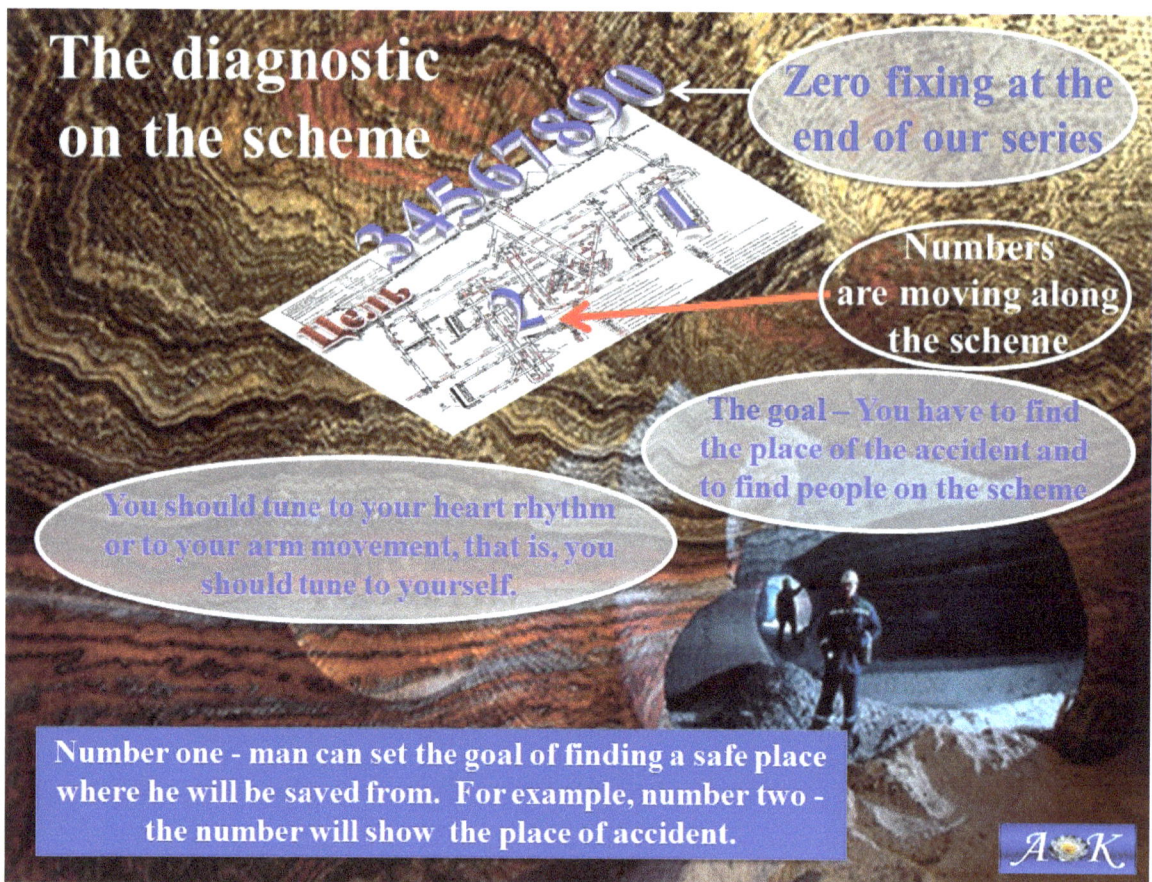

The diagnostic on the scheme

Zero fixing at the end of our series

Numbers are moving along the scheme

The goal – You have to find the place of the accident and to find people on the scheme

You should tune to your heart rhythm or to your arm movement, that is, you should tune to yourself.

Number one - man can set the goal of finding a safe place where he will be saved from. For example, number two - the number will show the place of accident.

12. The principle of exposure of number. Receipt of answer without solving the tasks on sequence of numbers 4798

In combined systems it is not obligatory to understand exactly the system, the main thing is to know that the principle exists and to realize it. The principle of exposure of number is related to external reality, it is simply enough to know control sequence. In work the situation is controlled at the level of simple logical phase of Consciousness.

Control principle lies in transferring the number into optical phase of perception. Selection of numbers is given by the Author of the Teachings. Depending on the task of control over these numbers you should bend out the sphere of perception into the spheroidal level, in other words we should as if bend a number series at required point of perception. Then both macro salvation and private task are implemented at the same time. That is, the principle of combination takes place here. Here the number is a macro control, and the number is a private task.

Let's take four numbers – four, seven, nine, and eight – and place these numbers vertically from bottom upwards approximately fifty centimetres from yourself and put the principle of goal control into nine. *"And place number nine against these selected numbers so that number nine was placed as close in the space of your perception to number four as possible".*

Control is: you caught number four with a sea line and pull through the top of nine, through circle, and at the same time number four entails the rest of numbers. You add torn structure of number nine to eight, fix control goal where macro level and logical level are combined in one task.

Testing of this method is presented in the second volume of G.P. Grabovoi's book "The Practice of Control. The Way of Salvation", pp. 284-286 – mine diagnostics, pp. 372-373 – answers to tasks without solution. After number four with the whole series was introduced **inside** nine, solution becomes visible behind nine in vertical plane.

"Control goal is to receive solution of task without solving the task. So, you must determine the plane in perception which denotes this control. And then you must see in space of perception: behind number nine place vertically a slightly lighting plane with weak lighting and simply perceive the answer".

Receipt of answer without solving the tasks on control sequence of numbers 4798

4798
Control sequence

Here the number is a macro control, and the number is a private task.

Number nine is place as close in the space of your perception to number four as possible

The plane of solution

to put the principle of goal control into nine

We should as if bend a number series at required point of perception. Then both macro salvation and private task are implemented at the same time

The sphere of probable solutions or the area of work is limited by plane behind number nine. This plane may be varied and moved in space of perception by more or less than two centimetres behind nine. We declare that plane where we receive the answer is exactly more or less than two centimetres – then we receive adaptation of this system on the system of future events. When we began to explain this method we told:

"the principle of number exposure, the principle of reviewing of number movement is the principle which resolves itself to work in accordance with the level which correlates with external reality".

This method is applied in the case when you have a task to receive a certain number, time or when you need a certain control system connected with the number.

13. The principle of exposure of number. Speed characteristic of number four

The method also belongs to logical phase of control which takes place at the expense of provision of dynamics to the number in development of own thinking. The number acquires speed characteristics – then we receive access of the number from the point of view of future processes.

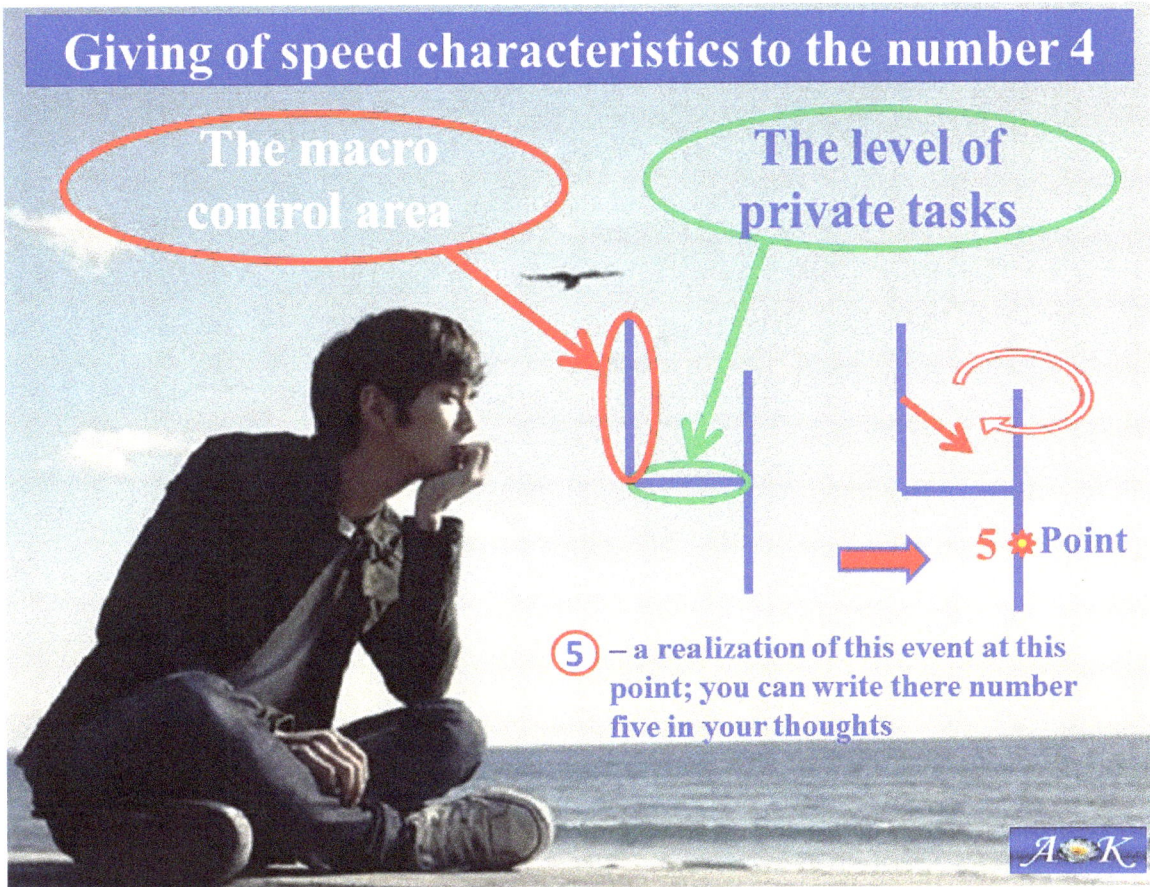

Giving of speed characteristics to the number 4

The macro control area

The level of private tasks

5 Point

(5) – a realization of this event at this point; you can write there number five in your thoughts

The method is represented in the seminar on the certain example of answer obtaining *"in the range from ten raised to the negative sixth power to ten raised to the sixth power – this is the order of migration"*. It turns out *"that the method can give preciseness in control and in access to information, that is, it can give certain characteristics of control even in case of great deal of information"*. The protocol from page three hundred and eighty four of the second volume of book "The Practice of Control. The Way of Salvation" is given in the seminar.

Grigori Petrovich separated number in the task of determination of migration degree – ten raised to the sixth power per second. That was the order of migration, though it could be any other, that is, there were no certain characteristics.

The core of control lies in giving of speed characteristics to the number, I mean, it is necessary to create for the certain number a path of motion into necessary point of control. As it is offered in the seminar, we separate number four and work only with one number. We review number four consisting of sections: upper free section is the macro control area, perpendicular to the section is the level of private tasks.

We try to bend down this part with macro control mentally, but don't bend it down in reality, at the same time set speed characteristics to the number that are in truth visible simply on the vertical line, though it looks like a segment on number four. And it is enough simply to fix the number of the event at any point on this line. It is just a small point designated by number five along the axis: you can write there number five in your thoughts. And conceive that we fixed the event at this point.

"Then you perceive this threshold level through number five as a splash of wave. And this splash of wave is a realization of this event at the expense of speed characteristics of number development". The number starts twisting and straining after the event, and the event starts realizing. This is a very efficient system in case of great deal of information. It is possible to work in this system at the expense of speed without separating the volume itself.

In control through the number *"control principle is chosen: it is either dynamics principle, if the volumes are great, or static principle, if you work with any private control systems"*.

14.a. The use of principle of dynamics of own body. Correlation of numbers with parts of body

A simple principle connected with body dynamics is used in this method. You select the number relating to the parameter of response of a body to external information. One may distinguish seven separate possible systems that denote man as a whole. Let's denote hands and legs with 1, 2, 3, 4; 5 is a corpus, 6 is a corpus with a neck, and 6 is a neck at the same time: two semantic meanings are created, 7 is a head, it correlates with number seven.

It is necessary to give comparable systems to the event scene, that is, by transferring the system just like on the analogy into seven elemental systems.

For example, we have an event and we need to receive control. Then we divide any event into seven systems and correlate certain

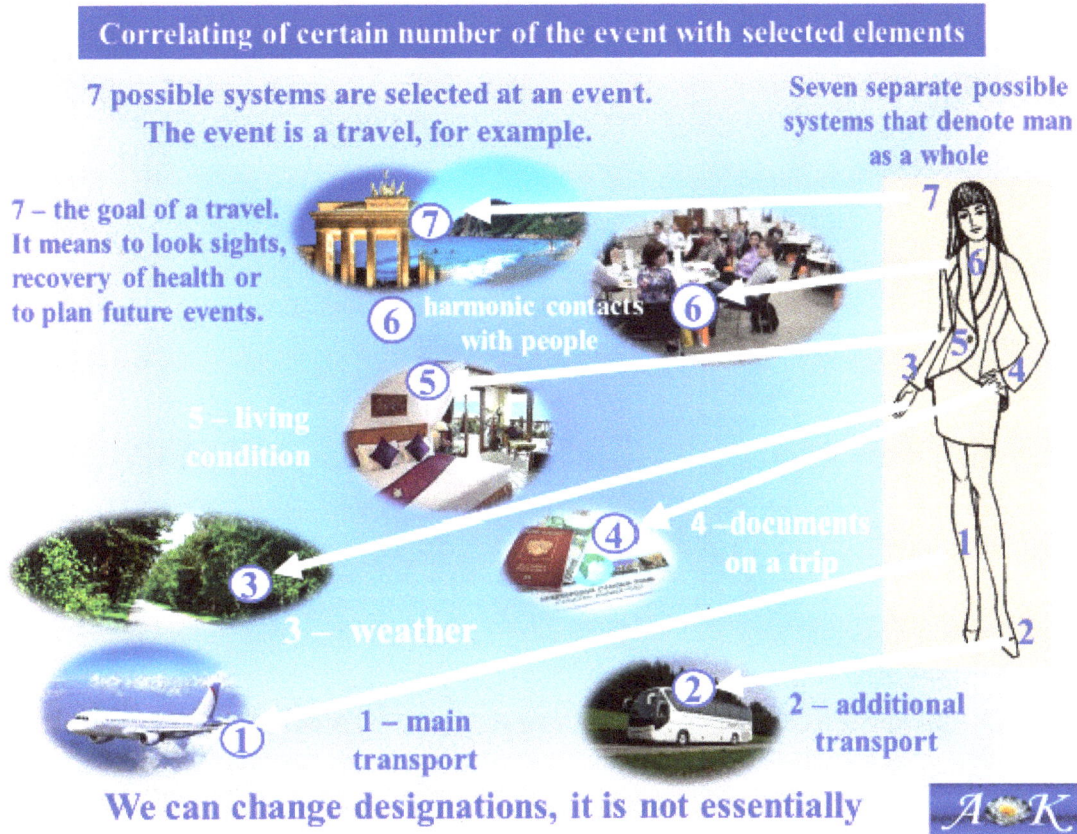

Correlating of certain number of the event with selected elements

7 possible systems are selected at an event. The event is a travel, for example.

Seven separate possible systems that denote man as a whole

7 – the goal of a travel. It means to look sights, recovery of health or to plan future events.

6 – harmonic contacts with people

5 – living condition

3 – weather

4 – documents on a trip

1 – main transport

2 – additional transport

We can change designations, it is not essentially

number of this event with selected elements. Whereby we can change designations. The scheme represented gives a clear division of the event into systems and control over the event exactly via designated systems of body.

There is an area in the event being controlled that we consider the main one and denote this area by number 7, for example. Optical beam from the head of man who makes control goes into the area of event under number 7 and highlights it, and the rest systems are highlighted by this area. We can designate any area as the main one in the event.

That is, control scheme can be carried out as follows:

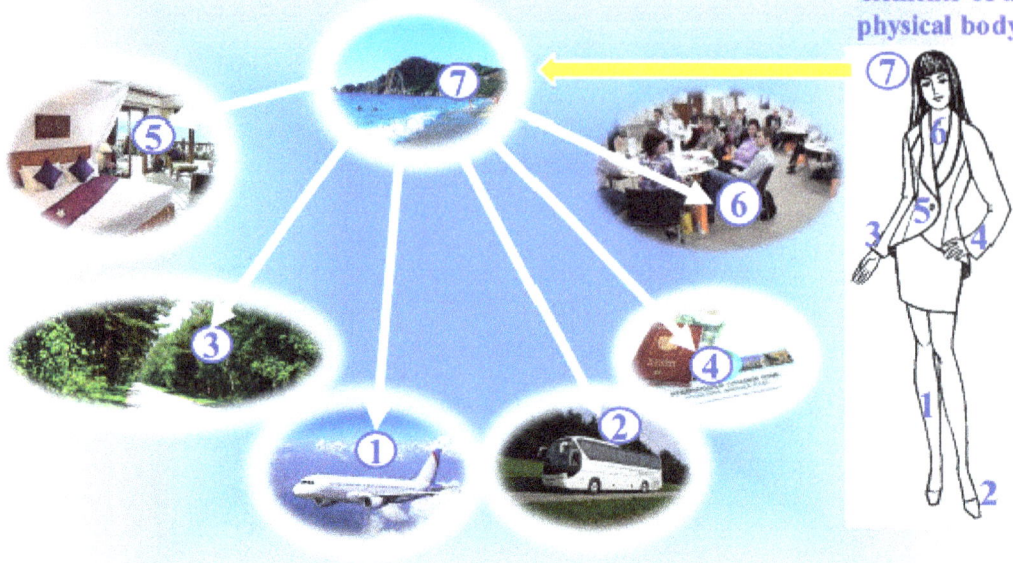

Control through a denote of the main area in the event

7 – the main event is holding meetings

The selected elements of a physical body

Interacting with own body, the man who makes control can work with the space of future to a greater extent

We can change designations, it is not essentially.

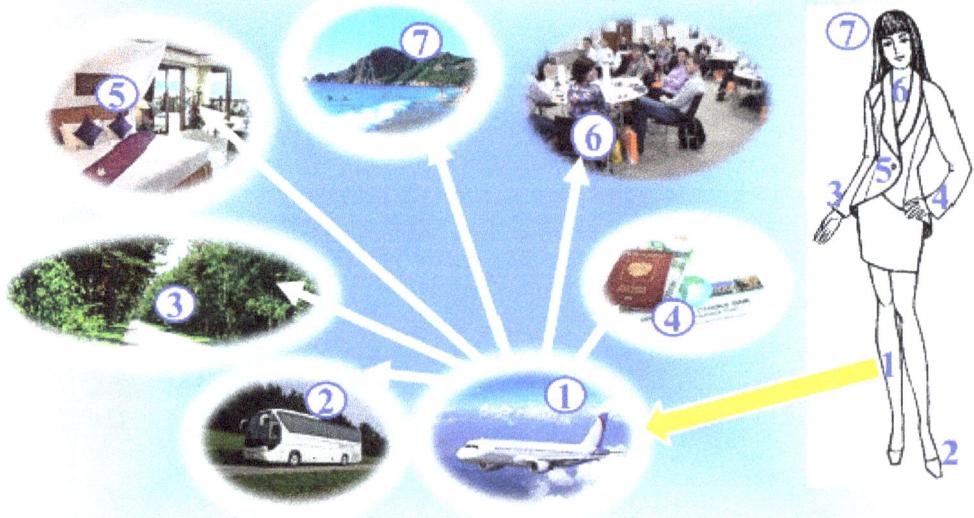

Control through a denote of the main area in the event

1 – the main event is end-point transfer

The selected elements of a physical body

Interacting with own body, you can work with the space of future to a greater extent

14. b. Work with the space of future through interaction with own body

When curing disease, it is enough to separate three elements, simply three fingers – index, middle, and, for example, ring, and divide the event into three events: diagnosis, then treatment, and the third element is recovery. Let's denote with figures and connect in thoughts each of three fingers with number, and fix it.

Fixation gives control only over numbers, it is no necessary to control your finger any more. At the same time you receive control mainly over the processes of future, because the elements of future realization, that is, future development are laid into body. Interacting with own body, the man who makes control can work with the space of future to a greater extent.

The author gives an example of inter-bank crisis forecast from the book "The Practice of Control. The Way of Salvation", page 411, volume 2.

When curing disease, it is enough to separate three elements

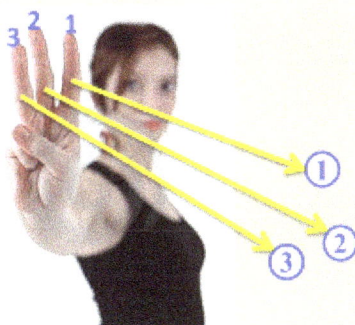

1 – index finger: diagnosis
2 – middle finger: treatment
3 – ring finger: recovery

It is no necessary to control your finger. At the same time you receive control mainly over the processes of future, because the elements of future realization, that is, future development are laid into body.

An example of the forecast from the book "The Practice...", page 411, volume 2

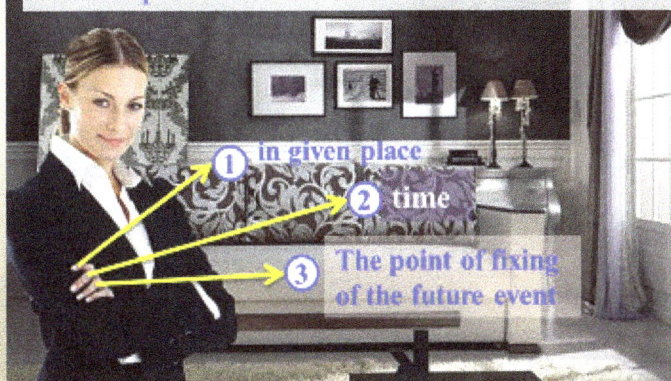

in given place
time
The point of fixing of the future event

1 – space "one", where the man who makes control is located
2 – the time till an event
3 – number three will go into a certain date at the point of fixing

Interacting with own body, you can work with the space of future to a greater extent.

The principle of control in respect of such level of realization lies in the fact that the space of control is simply divided into the space "one" in given place – number one where the man who makes control is located. Number two is the space of access, that is, time within which event realization takes place. That is, it is the time till the moment when an event will take place. Three is an event which must be given in forecast plan. The man who makes control works only with his goal, the problem of present (what event exists now) has very low attraction to him.

If you need to detect the control goal, for example, what you should tell to a certain man, then it is possible to fix this system on the same fingers again: one, two, three. And number three, fixed as if at the point, that is, at the place where it is fixed by the man who makes control, will go into a certain date. In this case the date is perceived as the level of number three fixing. And the control itself becomes simple, if man correlates it with the processes of the future. *"That is, the future is there where physical body of man works".*

15. Separation of macro control system inside the number for implementation of private task

In this method the system of macro control is separated inside number, *"and with such a high speed, that in any case your task is realized within such macro control".* You should go to this macro level of number "one" in thoughts and set the goal of control inside of securely fixed number.

Control is carried out at the expense of the fact that you admit development of events inside of a certain form in infinite area, that is, at the expense of infinity you anyway achieve control. Creation of infinity factor of internal area of number one is a mental and very strong compressing of perceived external level of number one. Imagine the number and start considerably compressing it by thinking, while the goal of control is placed inside. By compression of this number a ready event is extruded from this number. If you have two events, then it is better to work in number two, that is, it is better to work within the frames of designated number system.

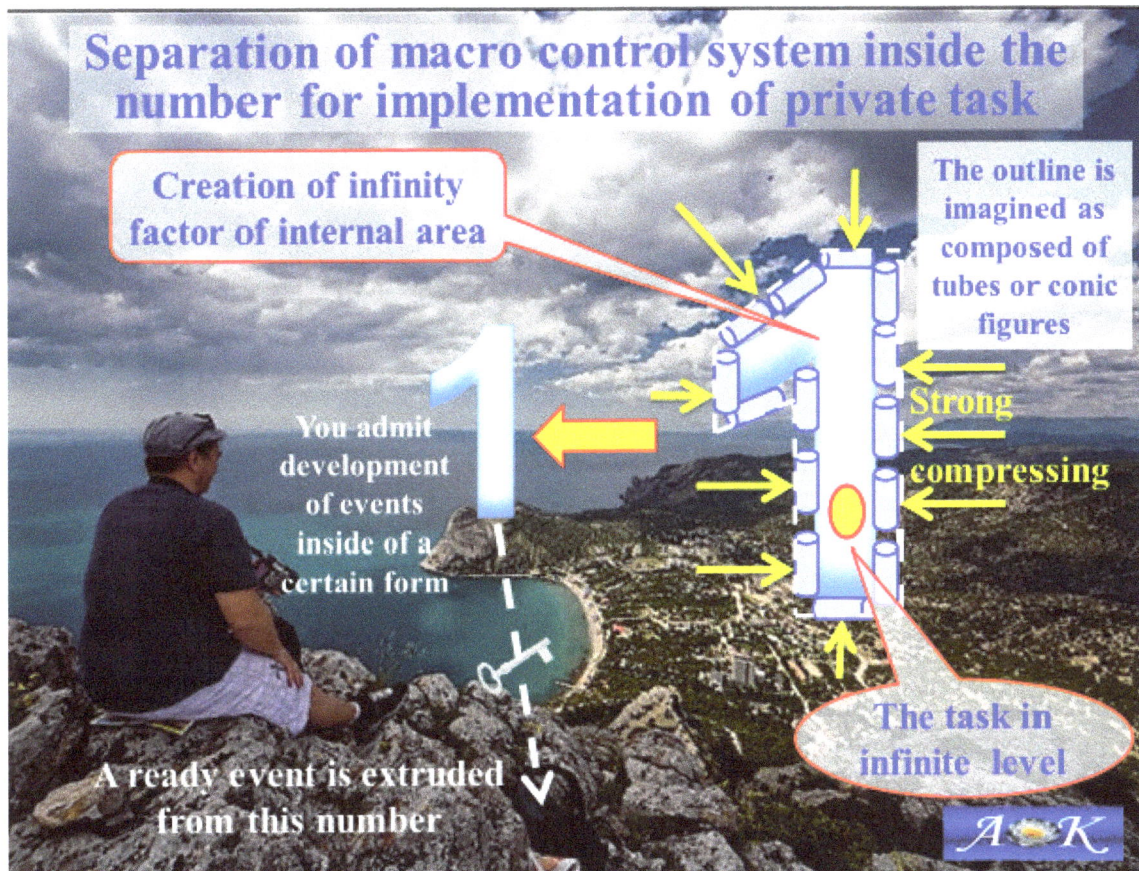

Separation of macro control system inside the number for implementation of private task

Creation of infinity factor of internal area

The outline is imagined as composed of tubes or conic figures

Strong compressing

You admit development of events inside of a certain form

A ready event is extruded from this number

The task in infinite level

As an example the protocol on page 437 of volume 2 of the Author's book "The Practice of Control. The Way of Salvation" is reviewed. Materialization of lost hotel room key is analyzed there. At the expense of Consciousness strain by conation a pressure was applied to the outline of number "one": the outline is imagined as composed of tubes or conic figures. The number shall be imagined in the place where realization of the event is required. In the example the key appeared in the bag where there wasn't this key for sure.

"Actually, this is the method where you organize the matter by the level, let' say, initial level, because if you want to understand what matter organization is, then overconcentration of information, yes?... some compression and overcompression give a material substratum. In this case the same technology is applied".

16. Creation of a number by means of interreflection of numbers

In this method *"the level of macro control and private task are just the number you work with". "In work with number series it is necessary, if possible, to find the situation when your spiritual development gives a chance to receive this macro number at the level of micro number, micro level of perception and so on".*

According to this method we show at first the number we are going to make control with to the structure of external reality. You can take any number and assign a control goal – and better from 0 to 9. As soon as you designated your control goal with a certain number, show this number in the structure of your perception: *"and this number starts realizing from the point of view of reality growth, that is, the next level of reality starts transforming the number you fix".*

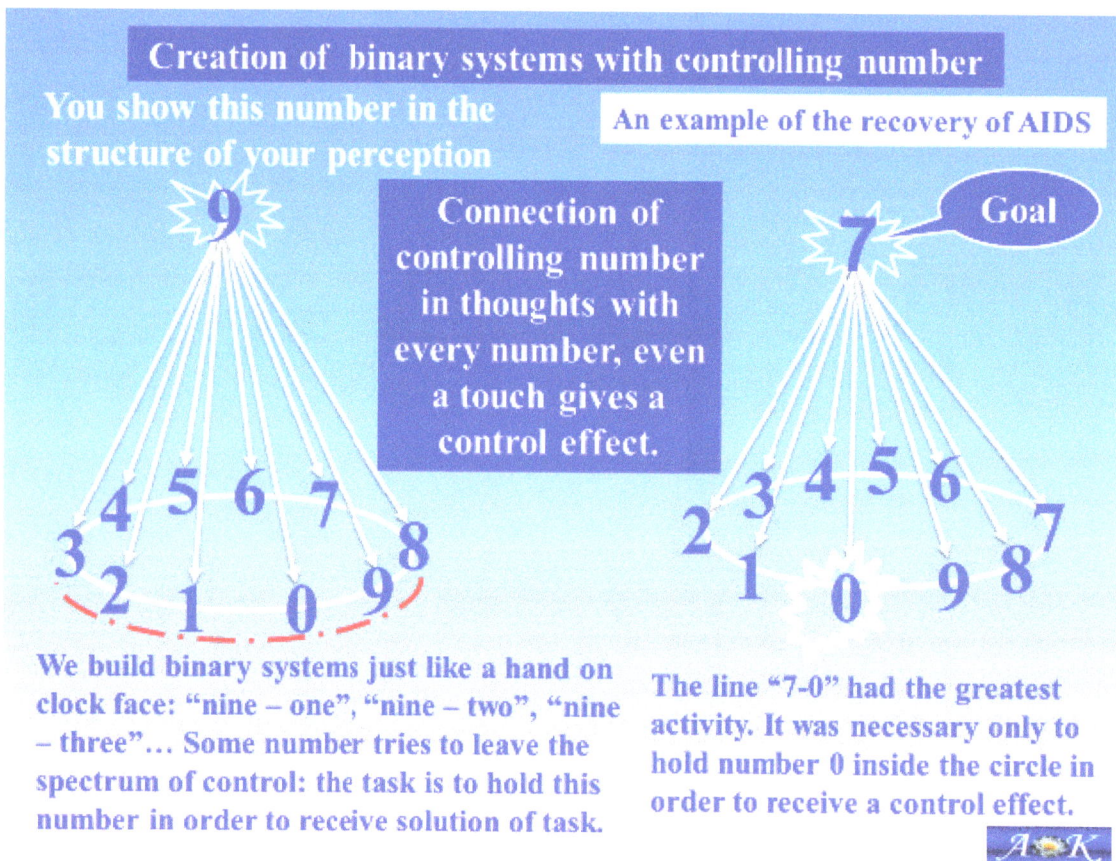

Creation of binary systems with controlling number

You show this number in the structure of your perception

An example of the recovery of AIDS

Connection of controlling number in thoughts with every number, even a touch gives a control effect.

Goal

We build binary systems just like a hand on clock face: "nine – one", "nine – two", "nine – three"... Some number tries to leave the spectrum of control: the task is to hold this number in order to receive solution of task.

The line "7-0" had the greatest activity. It was necessary only to hold number 0 inside the circle in order to receive a control effect.

To control the principle of transformation one should admit that the numbers will be changed, for example, around a circle. You determine the control number, for example, nine – that is, you should take into account nine parameters or you simply could like number nine. You place a control goal into controlling number nine, and put number series from zero to nine around this number. And then, depending on the shift of number nine, we build binary systems just like a hand on clock face: "nine – one", "nine – two", "nine – three" and so on.

For the method not to be too expanded and not to have uncontrolled systems of development inside number series, one can imagine a cone and from the top of this cone, for example, one can draw lines to every number. Number nine is at the top of the cone, we pass nine or any number denoting control goal over each line, then the whole spectrum of control is taken into account. Connection of controlling number in thoughts, giving of dynamics properties to connection with every number, even a touch gives a control effect.

Example of Grigori Petrovich connected with remote recovery of the fourth stage of AIDS (vol. 3, page 705): there was number 7 at the top, and the line 7-0 had the greatest activity. It was necessary only to hold number 0 inside the circle, and the disease was cured.

As soon as the man who makes control starts moving the number along the lines, some number tries to leave the circle: the task is to hold this number inside the circle in order to receive a control effect.

17. A series of spherical paths from numbers from 0 to 9

The method where you use the principle of closing of numbers on a plane: imagine the numbers from zero to nine on a plane and place a row of spherical paths.

Spherical paths from numbers from 0 to 9

Number two is setting of the task of macro control on paths

An example about recovery from inoperable pancreatic cancer

A controlling number two contains the goal of control in itself and it is in the level of macro control

"Homogeneity of separated number on two levels, such as spheroidical horizontal plus vertical level, gives a control effect", G.P.Grabovoi, 04.23.2002

You can put three or four paths, for example, the first one: 0 – 1 – 2 – 3, the second one: 0 – 1 – 2 – 3 – 4 – 5, and so on. Make one, two or three paths and set on these paths the goal of macro control in the form of controlling number which we simultaneously see on control.

For example, this is number two which can be imagined vertical on this sort of base – then we will receive a control effect. Besides the level of number two, all the rest numbers are separated in perception, *"that is, homogeneity of separated number on two levels, such as spheroidical horizontal plus vertical level, gives a control effect".*

The path is closed on a mechanical level.

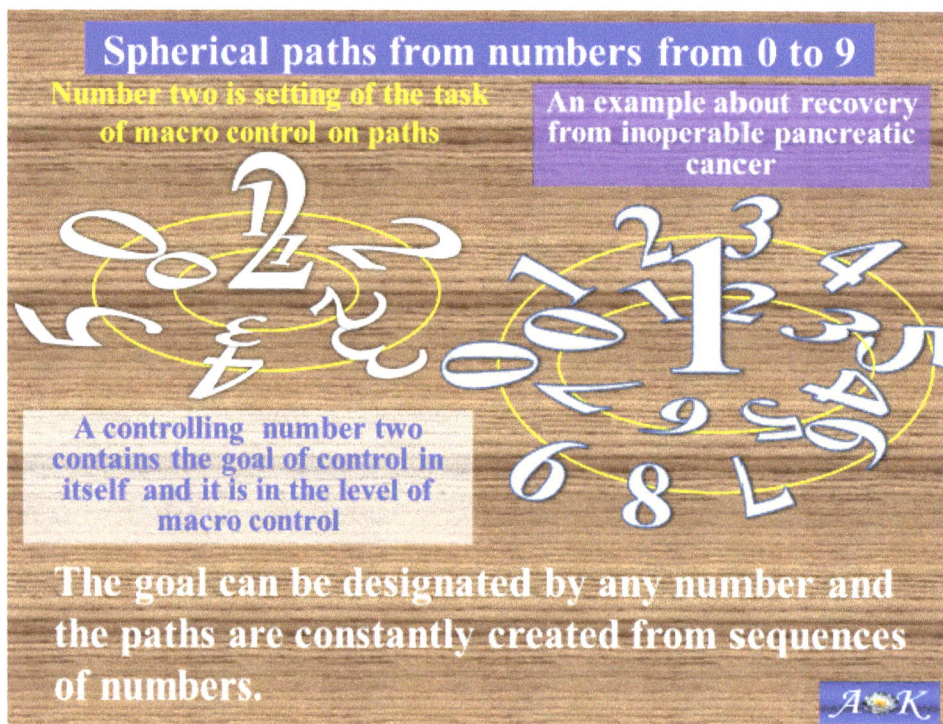

As an example the case from three-volume edition "The Practice of Control. The Way of Salvation", page 748, volume 3 about recovery from inoperable pancreatic cancer with invasion in dodecadactylon is given. The control goal is a recovery. The goal can be designated by any number and the paths are constantly created from sequences of numbers. The path is closed on a mechanical level.

"The principle of control must be so that you separate this number in order to achieve control from the point of view of stability and from the point of view that in truth you designate any system as a control one and you may correlate it with control".

CONTROL BY MEANS OF PHRASES IN EIGHT METHODS

18. Method of control by means of phrase on a vertical plane

Control is made on a vertical plane in the system of reference YOX which is approximately in 50 cm from the physical body in the area of perception, or it is possible to draw a scheme on the sheet of paper and make control looking at the picture. At first a control goal is formed in the form of a short phrase, then the letters are placed by sine wave: the first letter stays on a horizontal axis X, the second and each even letter form a kind of sine wave, that is, even letters make a sine wave, and odd letters are located on the axis. Take a usual phrase – "normal events" – and organize a sine wave from the phrase.

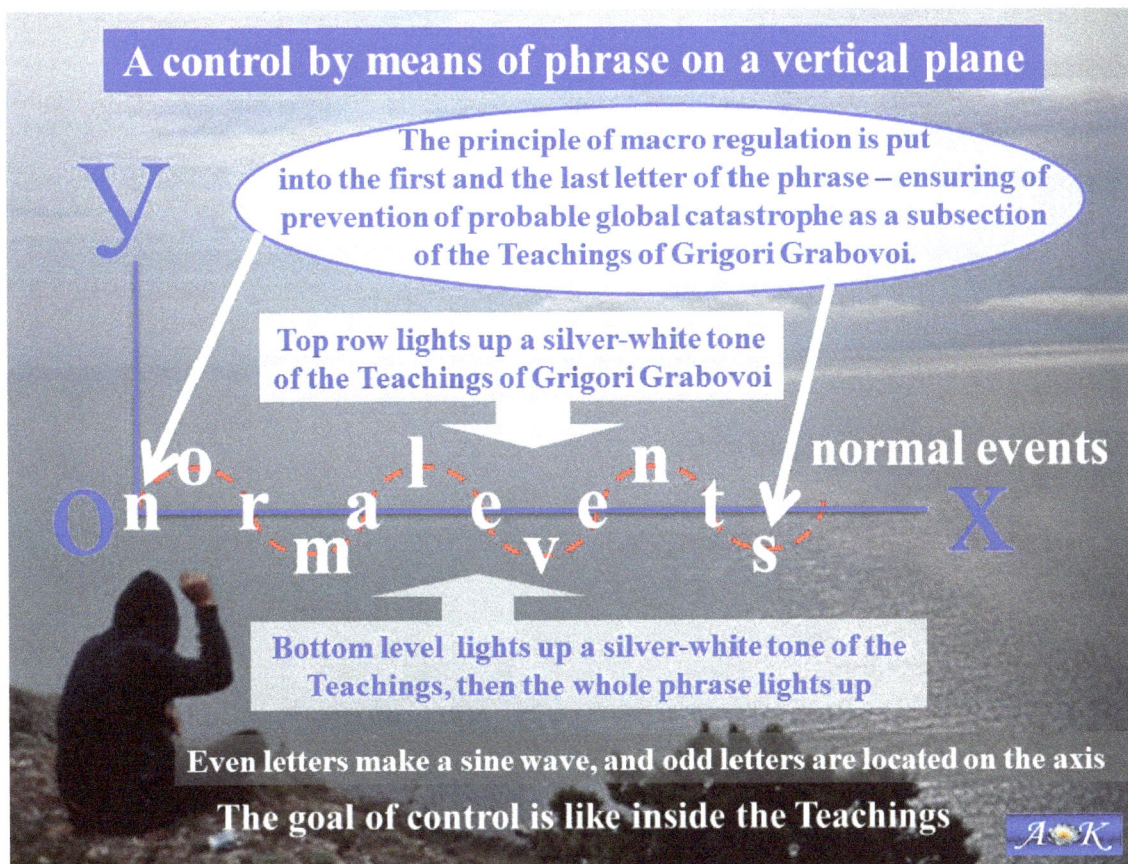

A control by means of phrase on a vertical plane

The principle of macro regulation is put into the first and the last letter of the phrase – ensuring of prevention of probable global catastrophe as a subsection of the Teachings of Grigori Grabovoi.

Top row lights up a silver-white tone of the Teachings of Grigori Grabovoi

normal events

Bottom level lights up a silver-white tone of the Teachings, then the whole phrase lights up

Even letters make a sine wave, and odd letters are located on the axis

The goal of control is like inside the Teachings

The principle of macro regulation is put into the first and the last letter of the phrase – ensuring of prevention of probable global catastrophe as a subsection of the Teachings of Grigori Grabovoi. So, the area of prevention of probable global catastrophe is not an abstract area but a substructure of the certain Author's Teachings. Logical principle of control is to enter into synchronization with the elements of usual optical distribution of information, while man organizes a kind of wave, let's say, from the control phrase.

The next action is to highlight the letters with the help of conation by giving them a silver-white tone: that is, to highlight vertically top and bottom levels of conventional sine wave. You can make control by correct highlighting of just only one or two letters: it is not obligatory to highlight all the letters.

"If you want to make control in the problem which is saturated, then you should actually from the beginning of this sentence, where the goal is formulated, go at first from left to right as if along the sine wave along all the letters, and then visa versa – from right to left. And in such a way you will have adequately highlighted controlling series consisting of letters, but at a far distance from you".

19. Method of control by means of phrase on a horizontal plane

The control is similar to the previous method, but the phrase is constructed on a horizontal plane in the system of reference XOZ.

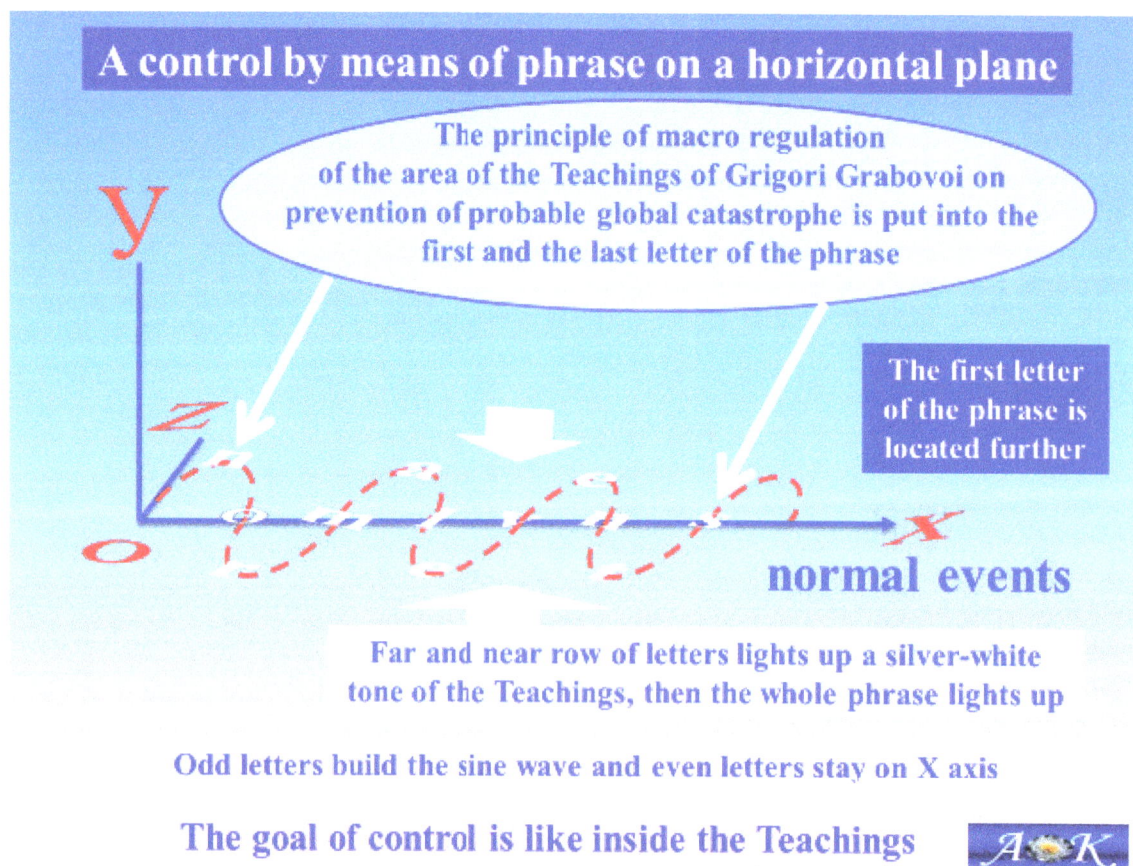

A control by means of phrase on a horizontal plane

The principle of macro regulation of the area of the Teachings of Grigori Grabovoi on prevention of probable global catastrophe is put into the first and the last letter of the phrase

The first letter of the phrase is located further

normal events

Far and near row of letters lights up a silver-white tone of the Teachings, then the whole phrase lights up

Odd letters build the sine wave and even letters stay on X axis

The goal of control is like inside the Teachings

The principle of control by this method consists of the following steps:

❖ The goal in the form of phrase is formed and written down the paper or in thoughts in the space of control.

❖ The first and the last letters are highlighted by the area of the Teachings of Grigori Grabovoi on prevention of probable global catastrophe so that not to search for the way of macro control, but to have a ready stable control method.

❖ The first letter of the phrase is located further, that is, odd letters build the sine wave and even letters stay on X axis. The movement of control is made from left to right.

❖ Then at first the letters that departed from X axis are highlighted. If highlighting takes place from one letter, do it from one letter, don't extend control. *"That is, in control system, you should bear it in mind for future – and you knew it - if control is achieved by the beginning of action, then control can be considered completed"*.

❖ If control shall be made by paragraphs, you can take one control phrase from the paragraph. *"Although you can make control by the paragraph, but you will have extension then"*.

❖ The system of reference is one of the elements of control in these methods.

20. Closing the phrase up into the ring with simultaneous self-recovery

The system of reference is not built in control as in the previous two methods: we simply use the space of perception, an actual space of thinking where the phrase is built.

You write the phrase immediately: you roll it in front of you into a ring just like a cracknel. Location of the letters does not matter, you need to receive a kind of hoop which has external and internal diameter: you should receive a ring in front of your chest – maximum width of the ring on the basis of the vertical letter. The letters can be perpendicular to each other or they can go one by another – it does not matter.

Highlight this phrase to the maximum. The first letter and the last character, for example, a point shall be designated as the Teachings of Grigori Grabovoi on salvation from probable global catastrophe and here an infinite harmonious development is added. Pay attention that two principles, two parameters of the Teachings are laid here.

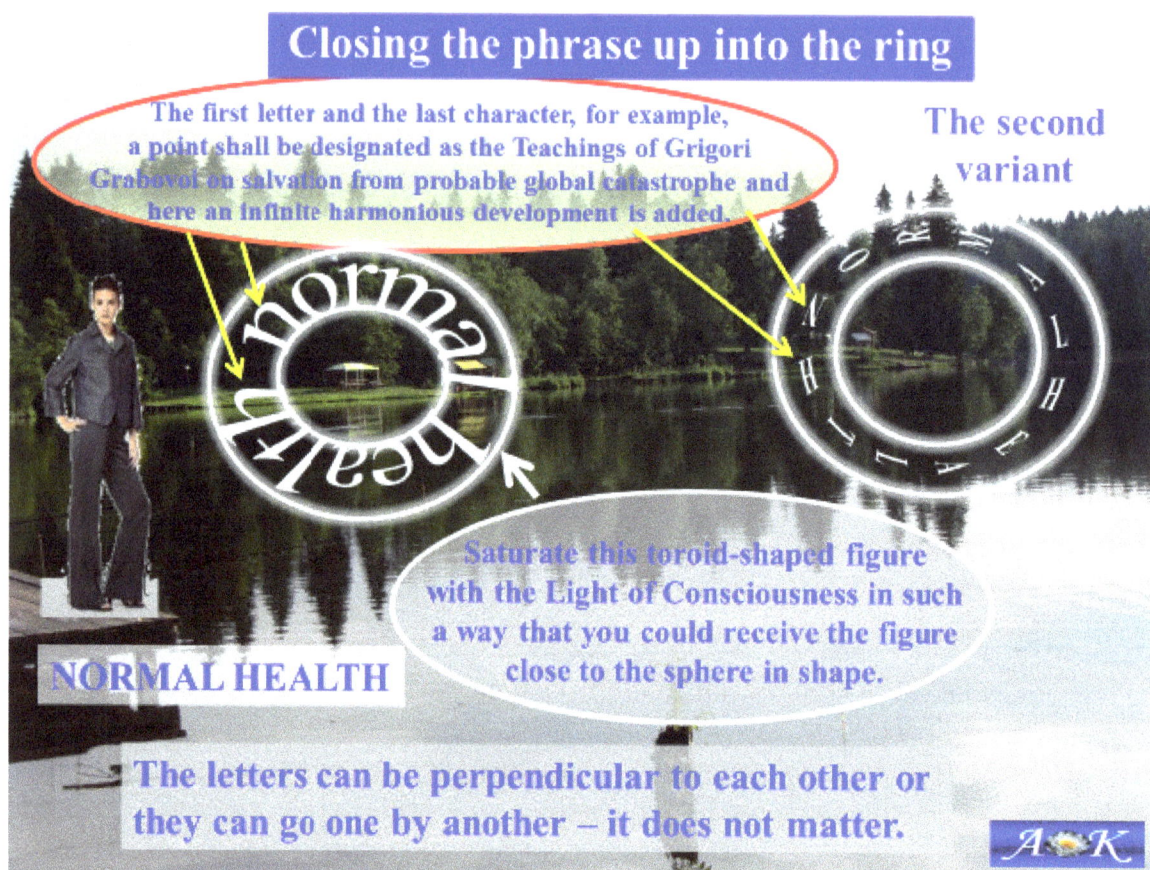

It is better to write the phrase on a toroid-shape figure not to have additional control because of formation of the other figures. Saturate this toroid-shaped figure with the Light of Consciousness in such a way that you could receive the figure close to the sphere in shape. The Light in the hoop made from the phrase shall almost have no difference from the Light of the circle itself.

Then you should lift the sphere approximately in five centimeters over the head and fix it. Physical action of sphere lifting over the head is the control action: you should hold the light over you.

When optics becomes stable pay attention that, first of all, it is the principle of simultaneous self-regeneration, that is, the Light of external control which you take to yourself, lights to you. This is also the system of self-recovery in case of action of the phrase on

Closing the phrase up into the ring with simultaneous self-recovery

5 cm over

It is possible the goal to set, for example: putting off of own fatigue. It is possible in principle any goal to formulate and thus to remove above the head

Simultaneously the person receives self-regeneration from the fact that he makes the positive solution in control goal and moves the sphere of lighting above the head

NORMAL HEALTH

"Any matter produced by you is also a self-regeneration in this system".
G.P. Grabovoi 5/14/2002

control goal".

In this method self-regeneration, self-recovery simultaneously happens due to the fact that man makes positive solution in his control goal and moves the sphere of lighting above the head, *"because any matter produced by you is also a self-regeneration in this system".*

21. Construction of rhombus from a phrase

The next method lies in the fact that the goal is written into control phrase and the whole phrase acquires the sense of the Teachings in the volume of prevention of probable global catastrophe – this is the first line around the phrase, and the second line around the phrase takes greater volume – it is eternal harmonious development. *"The whole phrase is informed with this control sense".* The first line is silver-white, and the second one - eternal harmonious development – is grey. *"You should start working there above the letters, do not start under the letters, because it turns out that middle phrase is the first line of division space".*

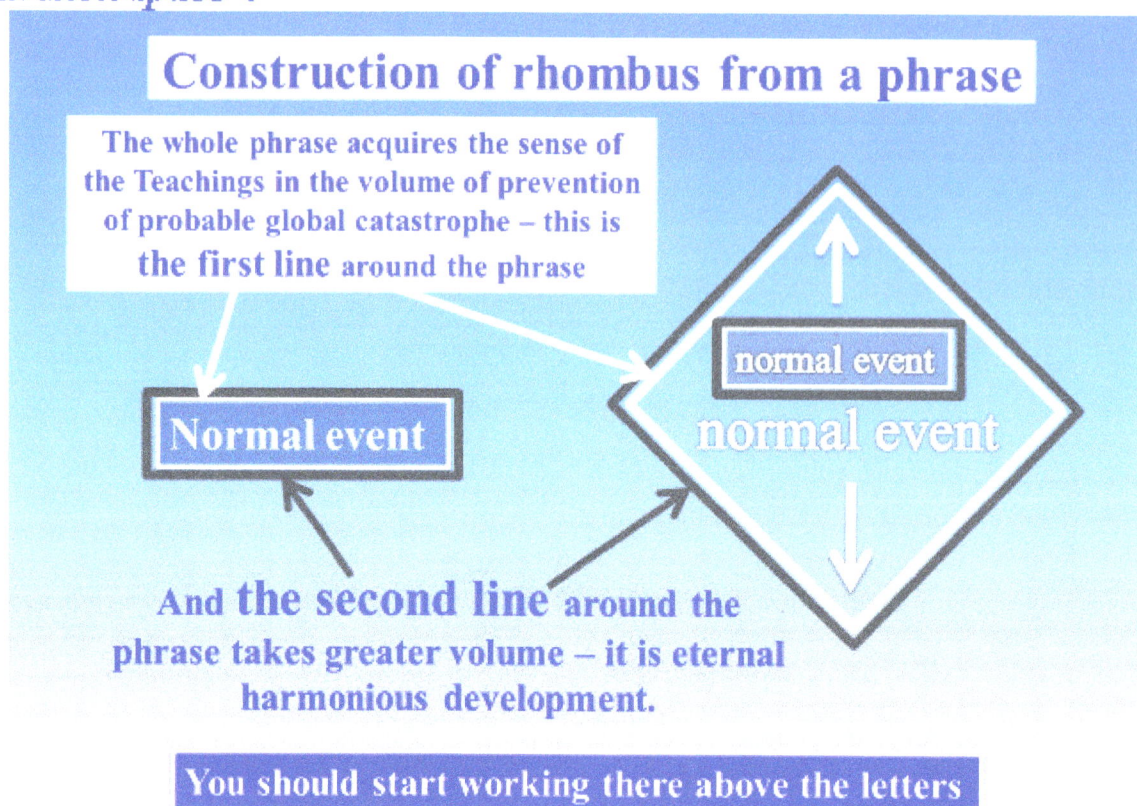

Construction of rhombus from a phrase

The whole phrase acquires the sense of the Teachings in the volume of prevention of probable global catastrophe – this is **the first line** around the phrase

Normal event

normal event

normal event

And **the second line** around the phrase takes greater volume – it is eternal harmonious development.

You should start working there above the letters

Then open out the space around the phrase and you will receive the rhombus. Deep in control you may receive control information: the letters will start forming into something like a special system of recommendations – what you shall do there.

"That is, you can build the next phrase further. That is, the next control is built behind the first level. I mean the next phrase – open out the horizon again up and down and so on – and reach a stable point. A stable point has the shape of just a little lighting sphere. And as soon as you reach it, it means that control in this cycle is over".

Pay attention that a new structure of reality is built behind the first control phrase. The deeper man goes inside the control, the further from himself, the brighter the Light becomes, and the stronger self-regeneration is: the Light from there goes to the man who makes control and optical lines may be directed to the place that should be recovered.

"If you need to continue the control: create the phrase again and go inside the control system again". The more man improves in control over this system, the greater the Light of peculiar knowledge and the greater the Light of controls is reflected on him.

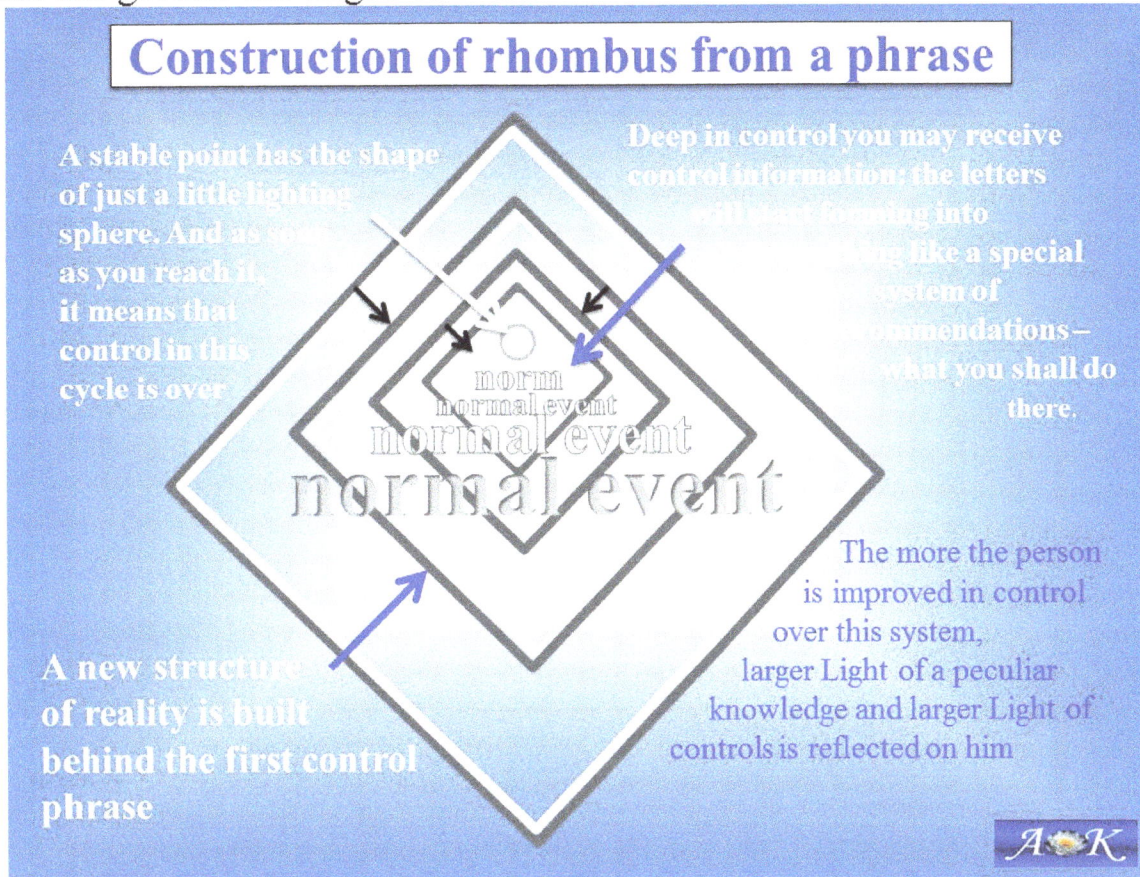

Construction of rhombus from a phrase

A stable point has the shape of just a little lighting sphere. And as soon as you reach it, it means that control in this cycle is over

Deep in control you may receive control information: the letters will start forming into something like a special system of recommendations – what you shall do there.

norm
normal event
normal event
normal event

A new structure of reality is built behind the first control phrase

The more the person is improved in control over this system, larger Light of a peculiar knowledge and larger Light of controls is reflected on him

A K

22. Phrase construction at the ring level. Spiritual control over phrase

The method lies in the fact that vertical phrase construction in the form of ring is used: *"it is desirable for letters to be levelled up along vertical plane".* There is no need to imagine a sheet in this system, the phrase is built in the space of own thinking in the form of ring without any base.

- ❖ Control sense in the form of area of the Teachings relevant to prevention of probable global catastrophe is put into the first letter on the left.
- ❖ The ring is twisted clockwise to the maximum. If control goal is very short, then the distance between the letters is

greater to receive a circle where the letters do not stick together.

❖ At the moment of twisting it is necessary to close up the first and the last letter of the phrase for them to intersect at least at one point.

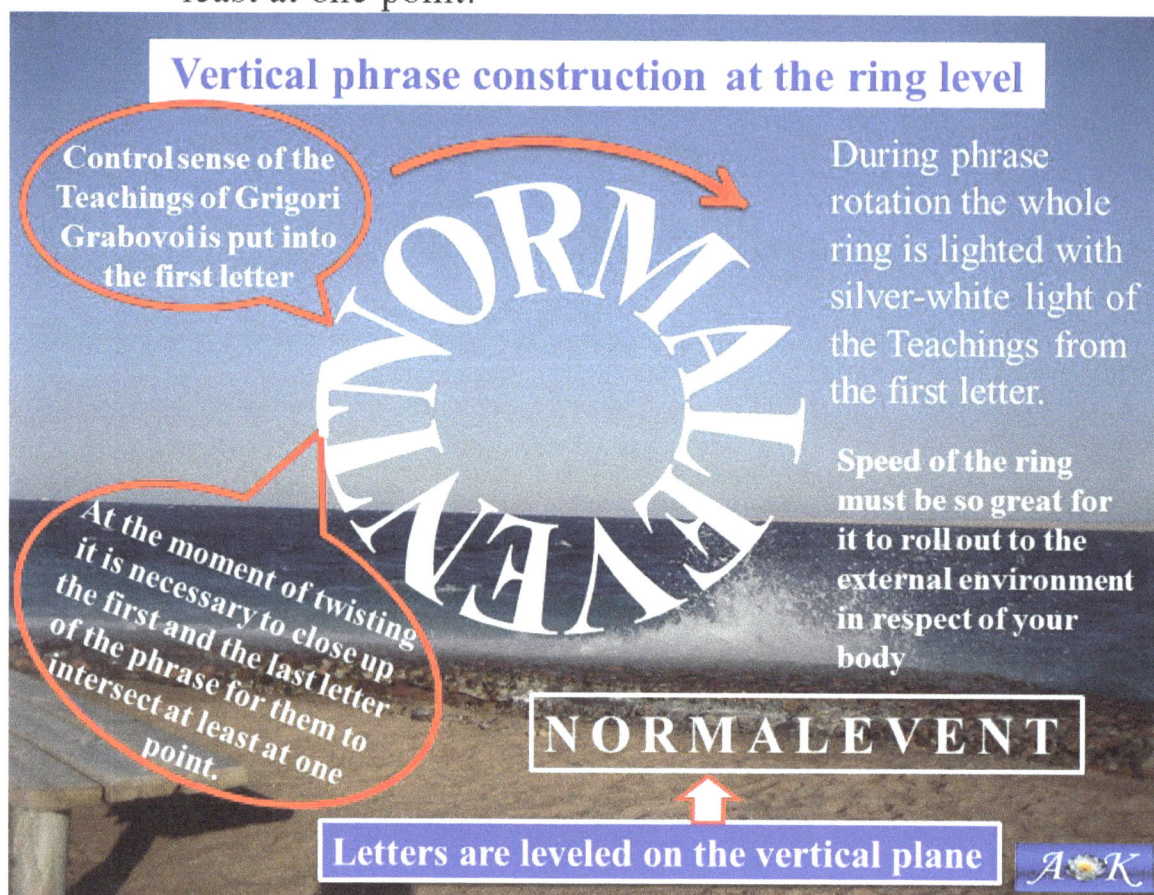

Vertical phrase construction at the ring level

Control sense of the Teachings of Grigori Grabovoi is put into the first letter

During phrase rotation the whole ring is lighted with silver-white light of the Teachings from the first letter.

Speed of the ring must be so great for it to roll out to the external environment in respect of your body

At the moment of twisting it is necessary to close up the first and the last letter of the phrase for them to intersect at least at one point.

NORMALEVENT

Letters are leveled on the vertical plane

❖ Try to hold the wheel vertically and twist, accelerate its rotation.

❖ During phrase rotation you can see that the whole ring is lighted with silver-white light of the Teachings from the first letter.

❖ Speed of the ring must be so great for it to roll out to the external environment in respect of your body, for example in fifty centimetres from you the ring rolls out, and then you should stop it with optical conation.

❖ At the moment of stop you will receive the level of spiritual perception. *"That is, you must receive spiritual state which corresponds to the goal of control performance, you get it?.. Here the wheel as if goes away into the future where you make control and receive spiritual impulse of this state. In this case it turns out that performance of control is put into the sense of this control".*

❖ In this case man must see in mind and put sense into this performance.

❖ As soon as the ring rolled away and stopped somewhere - control is made in the future and the man who made control received a spiritual state: *"what spiritual perception in this case is with this element of performance of this control goal. And then you simply fix the spiritual state. And this spiritual lighting is the control in this case".*

❖ Logical phase which helped you to approach spiritual state is also a controlling one, and it can be controlling in the first element, as soon as you simply designated the word.

❖ *"Achievement of the goal is often a uniform spiritual state in terms of perception, and in terms of optics it is often similar, but there are as many nuances as many performances of goals in respect of certain method".*

❖ Later it will be enough to recall and you will control in respect of any goal.

Spiritual perception with the element of performance of the control goal in a ring from the phrase

Speed of the ring must be so great for it to roll out to the external environment in respect of your body, for example, this distance is 50 cm

Spiritual impulse of a state at the executed control

As soon as the ring rolled away and stopped somewhere - control is made in the future and the man who made control received a spiritual state

"Achievement of the goal is often a uniform spiritual state in terms of perception, and in terms of optics it is often similar, but there are as many nuances as many performances of goals in respect of certain method", G.P. Grabovoi 5/14/2002

23. Phrase construction in the form of vertical ring untwisted counter-clockwise

The control method lies in the fact that actually during phrase construction in the form of ring man makes everything the same, but he twists the phrase counter-clockwise. The wheel, lighting and rotating to the left, moves to the right and to the left in parallel to the body, but not from the man who makes control. You can move the wheel even around the body: at this moment a pole of lack of access of negative processes is created around the body.

"This stabilization control is often necessary when you make, for example, a lot of or large volumes of work at the same time, and then you should carry out this control rather efficiently from the point of view of stabilization of Your control system for you not to overreach yourself and so on".

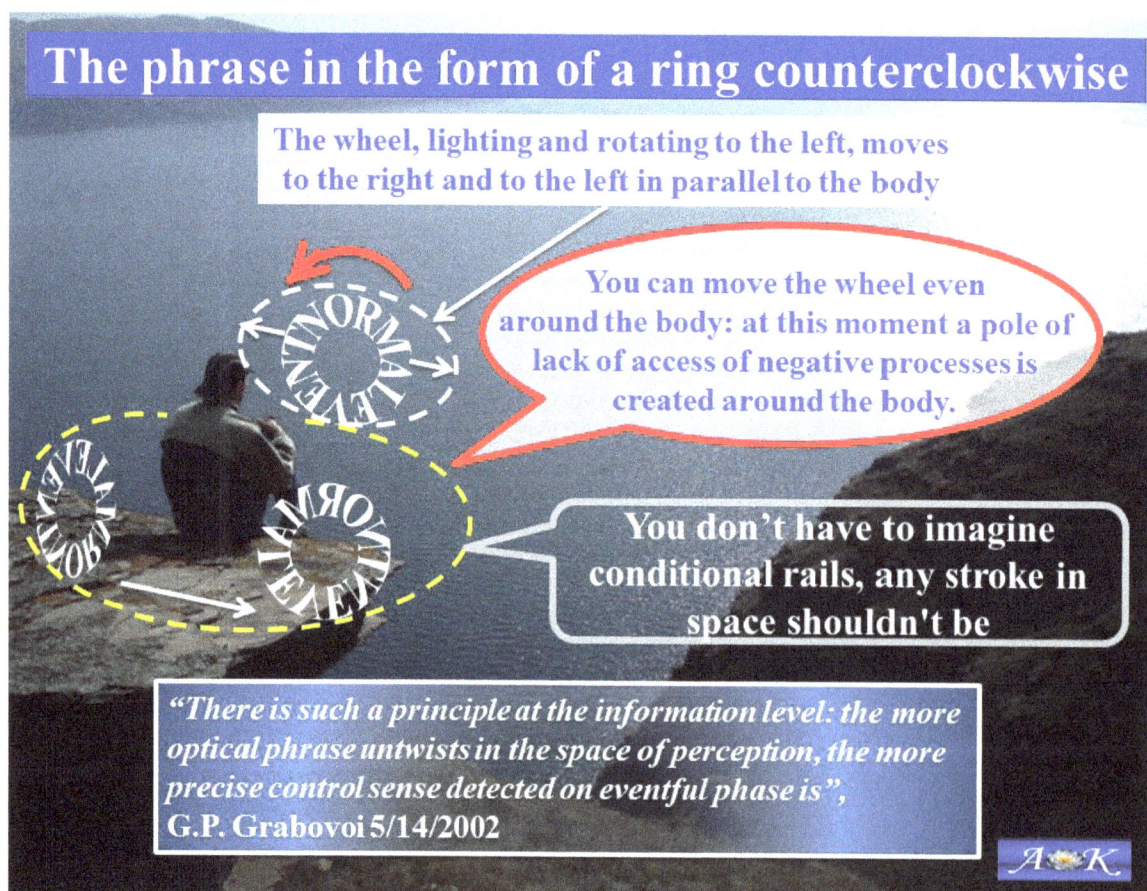

The phrase in the form of a ring counterclockwise

The wheel, lighting and rotating to the left, moves to the right and to the left in parallel to the body

You can move the wheel even around the body: at this moment a pole of lack of access of negative processes is created around the body.

You don't have to imagine conditional rails, any stroke in space shouldn't be

"There is such a principle at the information level: the more optical phrase untwists in the space of perception, the more precise control sense detected on eventful phase is", G.P. Grabovoi 5/14/2002

You can roll the wheel around yourself just like along the rails, but you don't have to imagine rails. If you imagine just a single line on the background of this wheel, control will become very inactive, because there is another medium down there, there is the medium of spiritual level. The wheel already moves in another space.

"When we make action, we create another space. Transfer from one logical phase of control to spiritual one is an action". When the man who makes control twists the wheel to the left, then a kind of path is created by spiritual construction. And then it turns out that spiritual sphere is strengthened simply by means of logical control.

Phrase movement is simply a logical level which allows putting any sense into the action, not only self-regeneration or autostability.

"There is such a principle at the information level: the more optical phrase untwists in the space of perception, the more precise control sense detected on eventful phase is".

In this method untwisting of the phrase transfers into spiritual control system simply at the expense of the fact that logical physical phase is perceived at the level of optics.

24. Receipt of light window at the expense of phrase movement

The method lies in the fact that control phrase is written in the space of own thinking. Macro control in the form of section of the Teachings of Grigori Grabovoi - prevention of probable global catastrophe – is put into three points of phrase – into the middle, beginning and its end. You can take even the whole paragraph for control, then you should find the middle point at random. Light up these three points; see how the light from them is distributed to the whole phrase.

Control: very quickly move this phrase or the whole paragraph vertically - up and down to receive light window. As soon as you receive light window – the goal is achieved. There is no need to do anything else in this method.

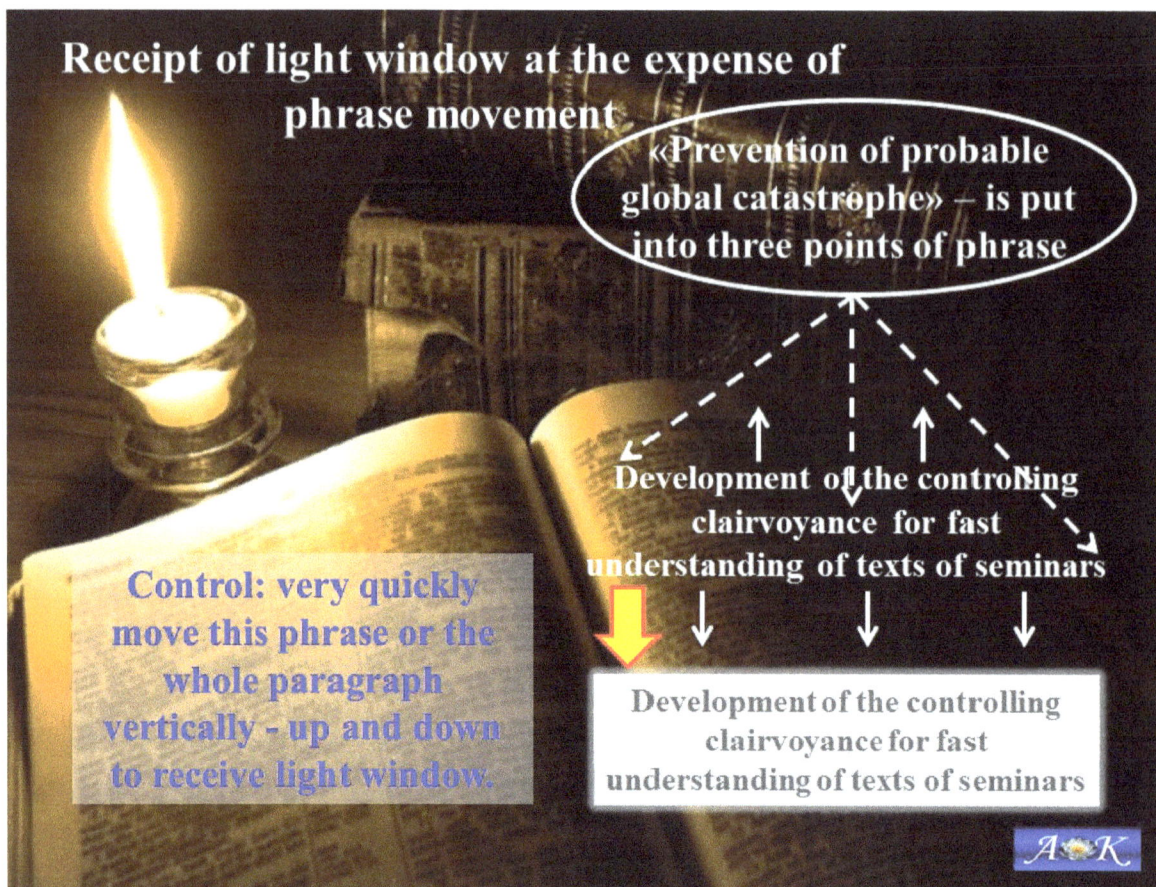

Receipt of light window at the expense of phrase movement

«Prevention of probable global catastrophe» – is put into three points of phrase

Development of the controlling clairvoyance for fast understanding of texts of seminars

Control: very quickly move this phrase or the whole paragraph vertically - up and down to receive light window.

Development of the controlling clairvoyance for fast understanding of texts of seminars

25. Combination of control methods through the words

The eighth method of work with letters *"is something like combination of all methods, their constructional relative position".* You may make and you may not: for example, combine the first and the second method, or the first and the fourth one. You are allowed not to use this method. Word or phrase is the form of goal in actual fact.

FIVE METHODS OF CONTROL BY MEANS OF COLOR

The principles of control connected with such aspect as color of perception is to minimize the number of control colors: it is advisory to control with the help of minimum number of colors in the first impulse.

Control is divided into the initial impulse: that is, control is made quick, ready accessible and efficient. The next level - color as characteristic of Consciousness or as characteristic of perception can be expressed as an infinite status: the color simply exists and that is all. It must be taken into account that even in restricted control systems the notion of color means availability of transfer of this color to neighbourhood area, for example. Let's imagine that a blue lamp illuminates into external space with a blue color.

External light influences control

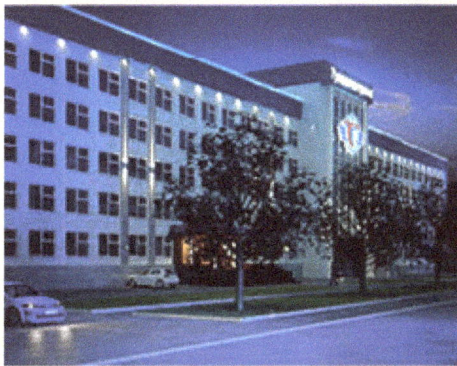

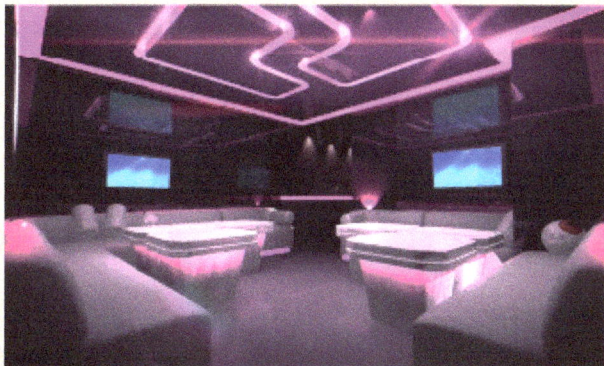

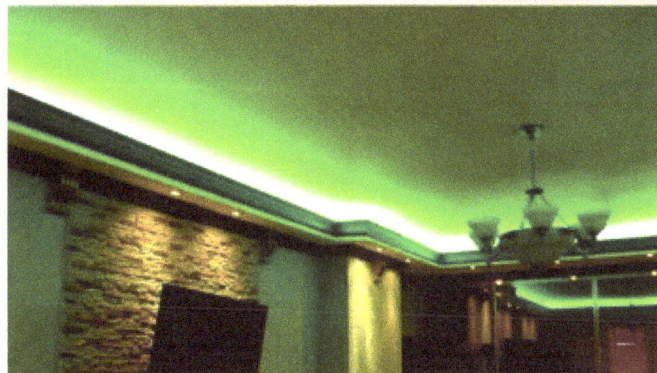

It must be taken into account that even in restricted control systems the notion of color means availability of transfer of this color to neighbourhood area, for example.

Fractions of color at certain levels can be intersected and it can also be a control element, that is, this effect affects the control. If you separate white and blue colors, then bluish, silvery halftones can be originated at interspace. *"In work with color such characteristics appear which characterise specifically immensity of expansion of color as a light, so to say".*

You can work with color in perception space where such rigid fixing like the one that can be characterized as *"almost like a physical space"* is absent. It is better to work in the system of rigid fixing from the beginning – it is almost like a physical one.

External light influences control: in the same way that we separate color in physical space, separation of color in control by means of color will also be at the level of fixing. When you work with color, work with initial feature of creation of physical space.

The scheme of control by means of color is as follows: the area of salvation from probable global catastrophe as a subsection of the Teachings of Grigori Grabovoi is separated in color, and further actions take place near this system of stability and constructability.

26. Method of control by means of three bent vertical segments reminding the shape of bow

The segments are bowed from you, just like you hold a bow in the left hand and draw a bow-string by the right hand. The first vertical line in front of heart, i.e. left one is informed by the area of the Teachings of Grigori Grabovoi. This area corresponds to prevention of probable global catastrophe. This is a line of silver-white color. The

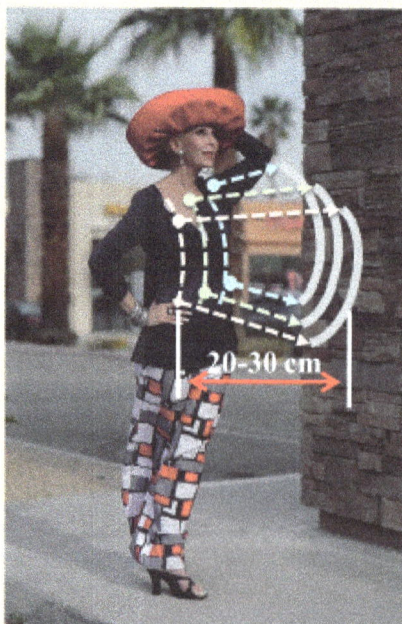

Layout of segments of a circle in relation to a body of the person

20-30 cm

1 – The first vertical line in front of heart, i.e. left one is informed by the area of the Teachings of Grigori Grabovoi. This area corresponds to prevention of probable global catastrophe. This is a line of silver-white color.

To the right the second and third lines – too have color similar, but they aren't informed.

Work takes place actually in physical space in front of physical body, for example, in 20-30 centimeters.

This system possesses the speed: and the structures the color relies upon, let them be light elements, have infinite speed.

All three bows are at identical distance from a body.

middle line is identical line, just the same one, but it is fixed simply as a color line. The third line is also like a color line. These two lines are not informed. Control lies in selection of necessary event between the first and the second line.

Control algorithm:
- ❖ Firstly inform, for example, hold silver-white color.
- ❖ Then select the other two lines.
- ❖ Work takes place actually in physical space in front of physical body, for example, in 20-30 centimeters.
- ❖ Take into account that access speed to this space is in principle infinite, because we talk about work with the light.
- ❖ This system possesses the speed: and the structures the color relies upon, let them be light elements, have infinite speed.
- ❖ Select two more lines, though it is close to man, but access can be long. *"It is connected with the fact that the higher the access, the more the space is compressed, compacted. The higher access speed, the denser the space is, because you work just like in physical space. That is, in this case space of thinking is very close to physical space. In this case you think almost in physical space".*

Principle of control creation from three bows

Event   **Similar system**

You place event between the first bow and the second one as if in a blank space.

Between the second and third bows the similar system – similar to the delivered event is located.

The whole control cycle lies in the fact that as soon as the first control system is built, you must start saturating bowed segments of circle with color. Color saturation is not restricted, but color must be light.

❖ Control is often made very quickly, strongly and as if in real time.
❖ You place event between the first line and the second one as if in a blank space.
❖ The goal of event may be not formulated in words, you can simply form it in a spiritual way: that is, at a spiritual level we know what we want: there is a wish, for example, to heal or a wish for something to happen.
❖ Here you may not fix the event firmly, but you should fix either optical form or to make more precise formulation.
❖ Place similar system between the second bowed area and the third one.

The whole control cycle lies in the fact that as soon as the first control system is built, you must start saturating bowed segments of circle with color. Color saturation is not restricted, but color must be light. Bows may have very quick access to any system – as though extremely remote or extremely difficult or complicated.

26.a. The use of control method by means of three bows to recover spinal cord functions in case of some problems in the spinal cord itself

For osteochondrosis the left area is saturated with silvery light – it is relevant to the area of the Teachings in respect of prevention of probable global catastrophe. The task of recovery from osteochondrosis is formed, and information about it is introduced into the space: and do not saturate anything. From the very beginning do not fix anything in the area of control except desire in the Soul or in the Spirit, that is, in logics. Simply consider information to be located between first two arcs.

Then start placing the next color – any color, you may place blue color, for example, as in the seminar. The third color is the controlling factor of dynamic control. What does it mean? Information between the first and the second bow – we think that it exists there, though it is inside us – place between the second and the third bow in fact.

As soon as you placed and fixed with the Consciousness – start looking for the color of the third arc if this process must be done. The process of control cycle often can be ended with the fact that we simply placed information between the second and the third bow – and control is completed. But if we see that control needs to be developed, then we start looking for the color of the third bow.

That is, the first two arcs may be fixed. In the structure of control via color the dynamics is high – so sometimes it is necessary to change static identification systems, for example, bow, arch, circle segment: they mean the same. When you start varying names, you receive a monitoring over control and oversee control in the first area, i.e. in initial one.

Example. Restoration from osteochondrosis by a method of three bows

At the left, opposite to heart, on a bow there is a silver-white color: the bow is informed by area of the Teachings of Grigori Grabovoi, this area corresponds to prevention of probable global catastrophe.

The recovery from osteochondrosis, information

The task of recovery from osteochondrosis is formed, and information about it is introduced into the space, and do not saturate anything.

We put the next color on the second arc, for example blue color.

We put primary information between the second and third arc.

We find color of the third arc and we control primary information between the first and second arcs. For example – we give green color to the third arc.

You can select a rigid form between the first circle segment and the second one, for example, the form of color drop. Because such a system at the spiritual level is a clear understanding and transfer of it between the second and the third level. Or you can separate light fractions.

In case of osteochondrosis recovery must happen – in this case it is simply a universal system, not necessarily a certain man.

You can select a rigid form between the first circle segment and the second one, for example, the form of color drop. Because such a system at the spiritual level is a clear understanding and transfer of it between the second and the third level. Or you can separate light fractions. In case of osteochondrosis recovery must happen – in this case it is simply a universal system, not necessarily a certain man.

"Diagnostics principle lies in the fact that these bows start buckling and transforming into more volume plane phase." You

may detect control achievement varying in the right part green color by intensity, you may also add some tones. The first principle is minimum: you achieve the first control goal, that is, recovery from osteochondrosis. The second principle: you may give details: for example, upper part of the bow is green, middle part is silver-bluish, lower part is pink and so on. We receive the principle of complete aligning of these bows, that is, only vertical segments are left. So, the goal was achieved.

The next control variant. Formulate the goal and introduce it the other way round: not as a spiritual fraction of goal understanding, but introduce it in the form of color.

Diagnostics by a method of three bows

The recovery from osteochondrosis

The similar system

You may detect control achievement varying in the right part green color by intensity, you may also add some tones. The first principle is minimum: you achieve the first control goal, that is, recovery from osteochondrosis.

The second principle: you may give details: for example, upper part of the bow is green, middle part is silver-bluish, lower part is pink and so on.

We receive the principle of complete aligning of these bows, that is, only vertical segments are left. So, the goal was achieved.

That is, it is possible to saturate interspace with color too and consider that control goal is color too, that is, control, but through the color. The task: interspace between the first and the second bow must be highlighted with gold color – it is recovery from osteochondrosis. Then, between the second and the third bow we must also place gold color. That is, we simply make two gold levels. And then control simply lies in reaction of the bow, which is placed to the right.

In control it is important to adhere to the algorithm:

- ❖ A row of certain bows are highlighted – three bows are in front of you: the left one is informed as the area of the Teachings relevant to prevention of probable global catastrophe.
- ❖ And then control goal can be immediately set.
- ❖ There are the times that once an initial segment of the goal is separated, the control immediately takes place. Then you are free not to give color because control has been already completed.
- ❖ This method is for not too large events, because the information introduced immediately affects the bows: for example, it is better not to imagine the spinal cord between the bows, because the action on the bows starts and control is protracted.
- ❖ As soon as we introduce the construction of thinking, we receive that the construction itself starts lighting and starts changing the structure of these bows.

The next control variant on recovery from osteochondrosis

Recovery

The similar system

You place a recovery between the first bow and the second one, as if in a blank space, in the form of, for example, golden color.

Between the second and third bows the similar system – similar to the delivered information, but in the form of too golden color is located.

And then control simply lies in reaction of the bow, which is placed to the right.

1 – the area of the Teachings of Grigori Grabovoi

"This principle of control from the point of view of composition of the system of the World lies in the fact that a similar element in respect to any system exists, and the fact that such element as a neutral system in a certain combination of event is also a control level. That is, such system is still separated here as a means of control, so in this case it can be seen as a control law".

27. Method of control by means of color – shields

The shields method is a more capacious system: it can hold many events and not bend. I mean that if you need to control over multidimensional information, then the method of shields is used. Some kind of shields bowed from you is selected as sphere segments. The first shield is closer to man, the second is larger, the third is the largest – it is informed with the area of the Teachings of Grigori Grabovoi relevant to prevention of probable global catastrophe. This is the control segment, control shield.

"When we choose semispheres we something like make larger volume of information, then we can highlight control system to a

larger extent".

The control goal is placed between large shield and internal segment of the sphere. *"In this case control goal can be viewed more detailed, more rigidly and briefly, as a light segment connecting center or any part of the first shield and the second one as a tube, and inside it all events take place".*

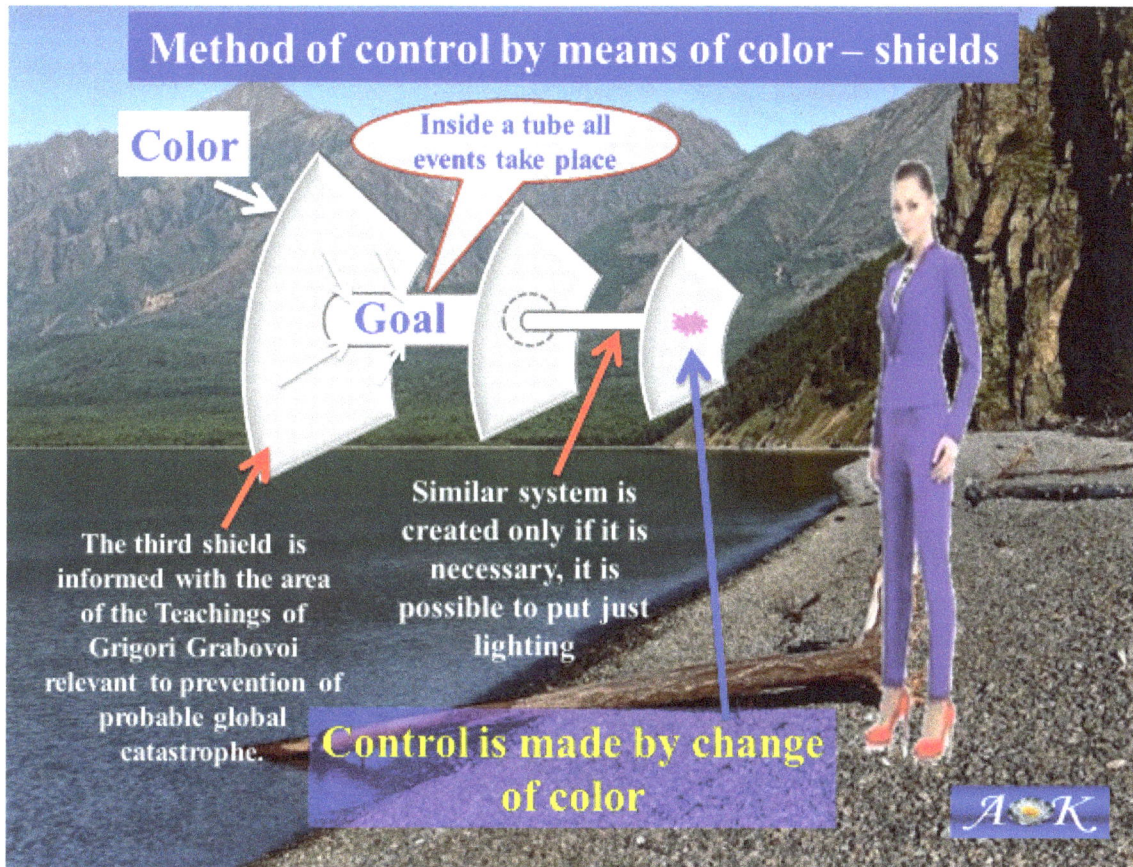

Here you also need to vary intensity of event demonstration in color and light aspects. Semispheres have a larger volume than bows, so they can highlight more information. It is just like in work with two flashlights – it is necessary to ensure that construction of events doesn't highlight the color of this shield on your perception: not to shade, for example. In the space between the shields one may place a healthy man or a nuclear power station. The system is very stable, it is not bowed, you can work for a long period of time.

The same event should be placed between the first and the second shield closer to man. Control is carried out by means of changing of the color of the shield, which is closer to you, as if this segment of the sphere.

Control can be absolutely local, that is to highlight one point in any place of semisphere-shield, retaining everything the rest of approximately the same color as everything else. Color in fact can stay simply silvery-white and control can be carried out even because you act this way: you use control laws through the color system.

The task is not to admit explosion of a nuclear power station: the one which really exists and can bring to global catastrophe. Placing this nuclear power station between the segment of sphere which is larger in radius and internal segment, you already make control. Shields may be considered as a rather convenient, always available pattern; it is a color any way, the light of your perception, and the forms correspond to this color or colors.

The construction is simple: information about the problem at the nuclear power station came into existence – you take and cast it right there in your perception. And that is all – there is no need to do anything at all. *"Then regulation processes start and they act so that such explosion not to happen".* If we think that something should be added, then we start working with the level of this segment of a sphere which is closer to you.

Then we should saturate the object with color. In this case each element is the control. Then we can create similar system: it is not strictly here – similar system is created only if it is necessary. In principle it is better to put thought – lighting, because in truth lighting of such system happens by strengthening of the light, and anyway it exists in the form of control – it is the state of similar system. During work with color in the Soul or in the Spirit color possesses infinite level of lighting, so you anyway involve, project the system.

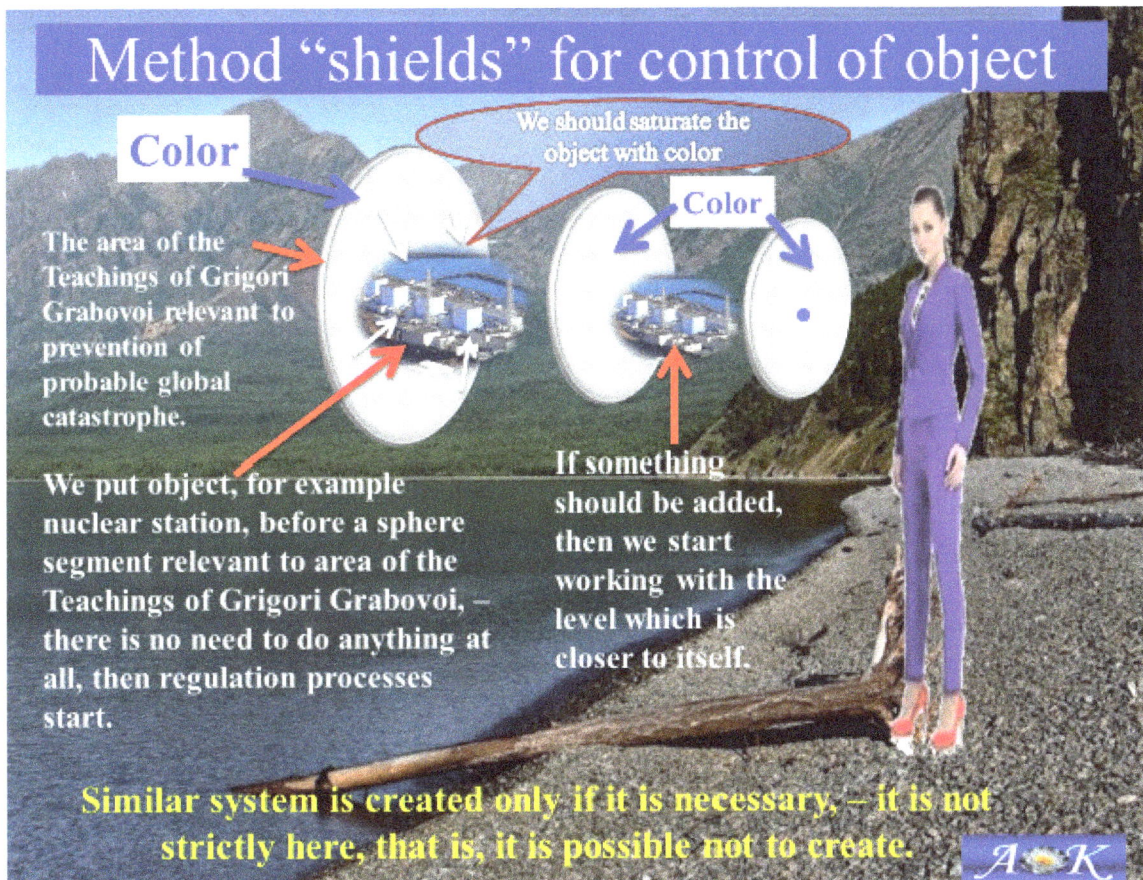

Method "shields" for control of object

Color

We should saturate the object with color

Color

The area of the Teachings of Grigori Grabovoi relevant to prevention of probable global catastrophe.

We put object, for example nuclear station, before a sphere segment relevant to area of the Teachings of Grigori Grabovoi, – there is no need to do anything at all, then regulation processes start.

If something should be added, then we start working with the level which is closer to itself.

Similar system is created only if it is necessary, – it is not strictly here, that is, it is possible not to create.

Why is the creation of such systems obligatory? Because it is the level of stability and the control level. You built the next station by conation – it is clear that color is not developed uncontrolled. And then the Soul and the Spirit work as follows: there are other laws of optical distribution of information than in logics, in physical World. It turns out that later you work on the basis of the laws of Soul, that is, it is the transition between the optics of Soul work and optics of work of logical phase of Consciousness.

Work with light is often a very delicate work, but it can be located right in control system. *"As soon as we create great volumes, they will have specificity for control over some certain processes. That is why during control via color you find the class of control systems, if it is possible, I mean that you distribute what is better at that moment: a quick access or intensity of control".* You fixed a nuclear power station for two times – hold it in mind for several seconds: then it is better to hold it on large volumes, that is, on shields, but not on bows.

And here you can also work with outline of the nuclear power station, plus an external shield – it is the same as a control board: you can highlight some positions, that is, highlight some points, areas with own Consciousness, you can build near this closer shield – if possible without interfering with two previous shields – you can build control at the expense of near color areas.

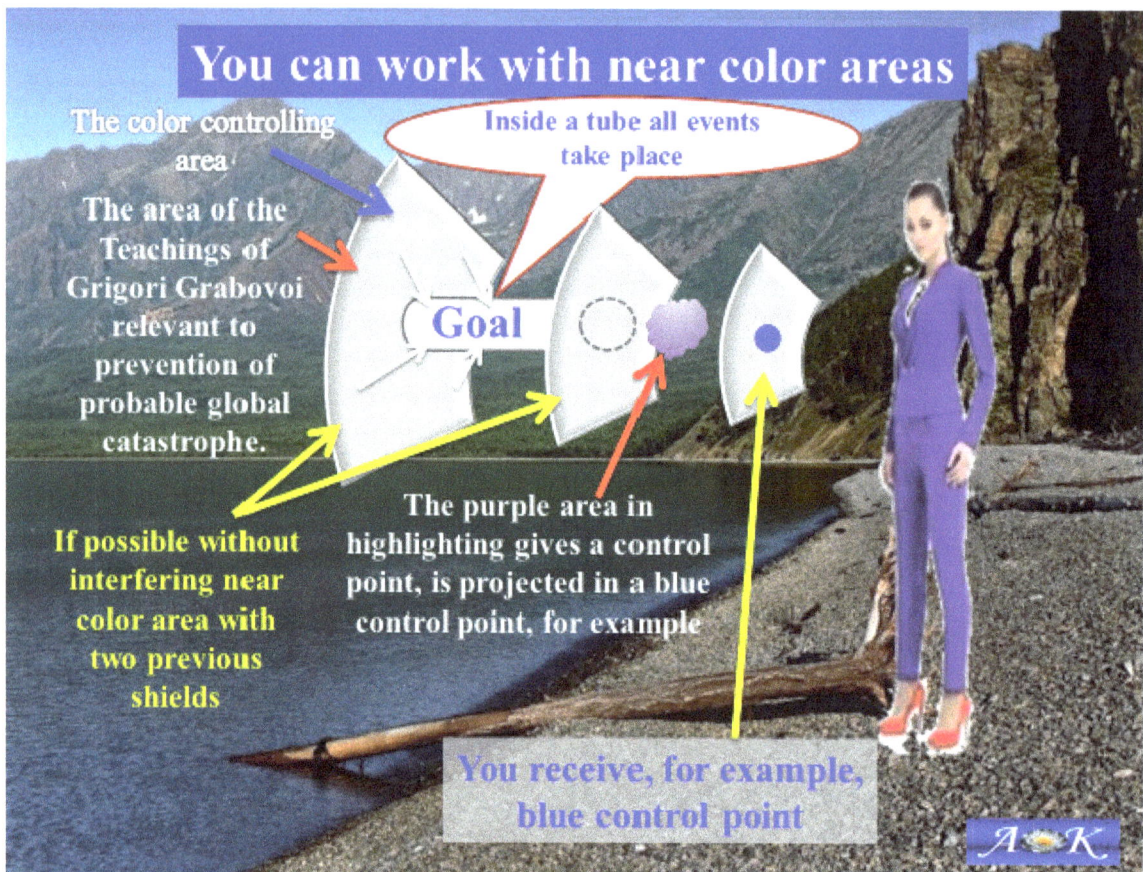

In control with color it is better to work at first with neutral silver-white color: and achieve control goal. Then you may start coloring – it is a minimization of optimality. You can work with near color area, and not obligatory in the system itself, because with color it is enough to vary control in terms of access and pressure force. By the way, it is possible to work just like on the weigh-scales.

Color control helps avoiding halftones, for example, you highlighted purple area. *"And the purple area gives control point, projects, you receive blue control point – it is not necessarily to be purple".* It is exactly separation of a light fraction that can be used here as a precise control technology as far as color wave propagation is a very precise system: simply because color always has a maximum principle of entry to the system. Maximum access is a controllability of control too.

"Characteristics of controllability are in functions of possibility of color itself which is a point of joint in this case of optical systems of Spirit and logics, that is, Consciousness". Highlighting of structure of the Teachings on the third color shield – disciples, followers work there – already gives prevention of probable global catastrophe because there are just the technologies that know this system.

28. Color spot method

It is a simple and available method at first sight. We build control area in front of us in the form of a color spot.

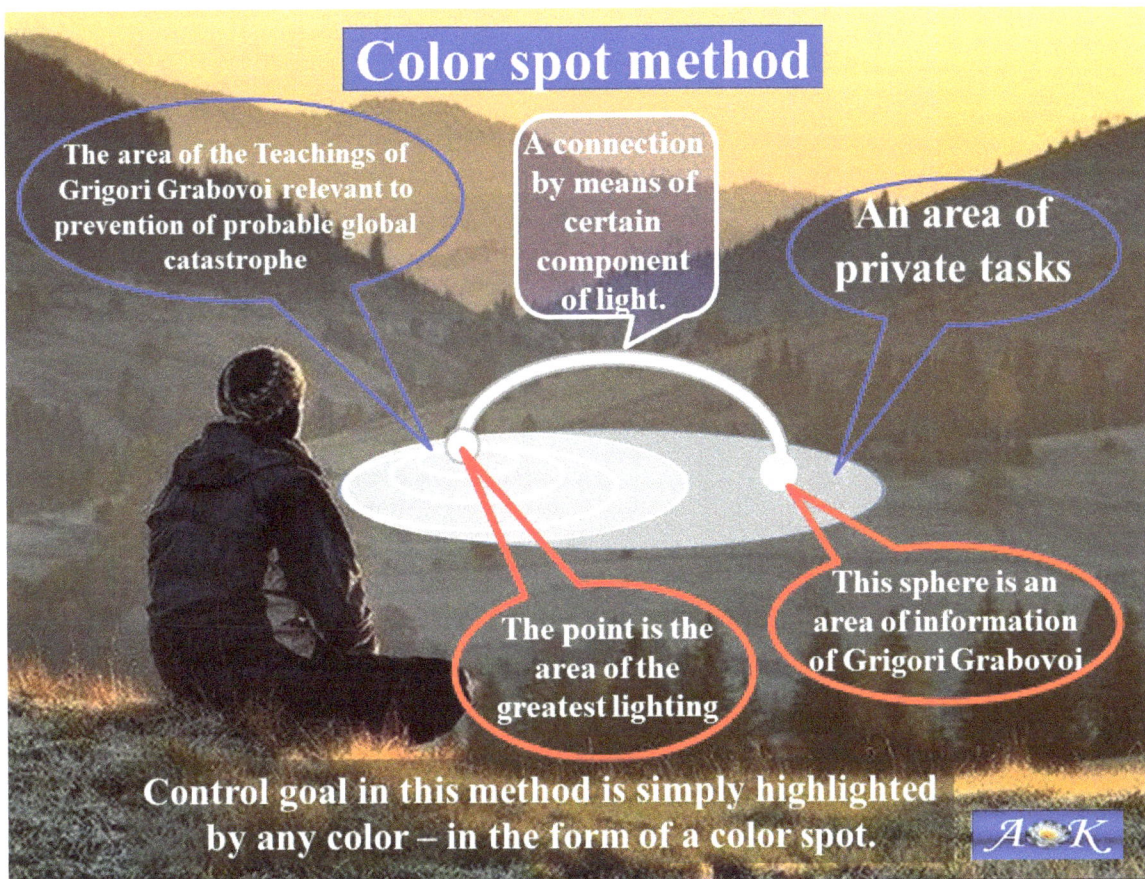

Control goal in this method is simply highlighted by any color – and any color is immediately designated. Approximately half of control area is selected on the left: and it is determined as the area of the Teachings of Grigori Grabovoi relevant to prevention of probable global catastrophe. In this area the terrain is selected – a surface which resembles the system of bulges into the area of conic development in respect of you. Find on this bulge a smaller area of the greatest lighting.

Control here lies in the fact that in perception – it is the sense, the fineness of control – the selected area of the Teachings relevant to prevention of probable global catastrophe must be highlighted to the left at maximum. At the same time select in the area of the Teachings the point which lights most of all: in its larger part it is higher, closer to us.

To the right is that what is called private control, that is, to the right an area of private tasks, private level of the event is separated. In the right part of control we may specify an area of information of Grigori Grabovoi – highlight it in the form of a sphere, for example. Control goal should be selected so that from the area of Grigori Grabovoi's information there was a connection by means of certain component of light. Applied technology by the task may act on control at once.

And then the most lightful components are selected in the area of the Teachings: the process of selection is already the control. And often it is enough simply to select something like a lightful spot in such a level.

Control goal can be absolutely different – these can be macro events, political, regional, I mean you can work just like with a map, an atlas of events. If it is like a treatment system – then man himself must be highlighted in the form of outline of a physical body: this outline is behind a light lens.

The work is carried out with silver-white color. Silvery halftone gives dynamics to white color, that is, instead of car driving speed a space velocity originates if white color is given silvery halftone. Grigori Petrovich Grabovoi analyzes in this method such notion as information of control – how does it grow? *"Because you perceive the whole World and reality in the form of color systems: light, colors... We receive information – in optical variant it is perceived exactly as color or light. Therefore, it is possible to work with very deep systems of the World in simple notions".*

"The next element lies in the fact that it is macro access, an ideological goal of salvation of everyone gives very high concentration in goal systems of control". For example, you see that prevention of probable global catastrophe has already taken place from the point of view of development of light spectrum, then you can

introduce parameter of personal salvation of everyone not to admit even a minor local catastrophe. It is in such a way here: you may control by the goal of recovery only by holding to the plan of macro catastrophe prevention putting the same plan into recovery. That is, when healing you anyway make the same work: not to admit probable global catastrophe and to provide for eternal harmonious development.

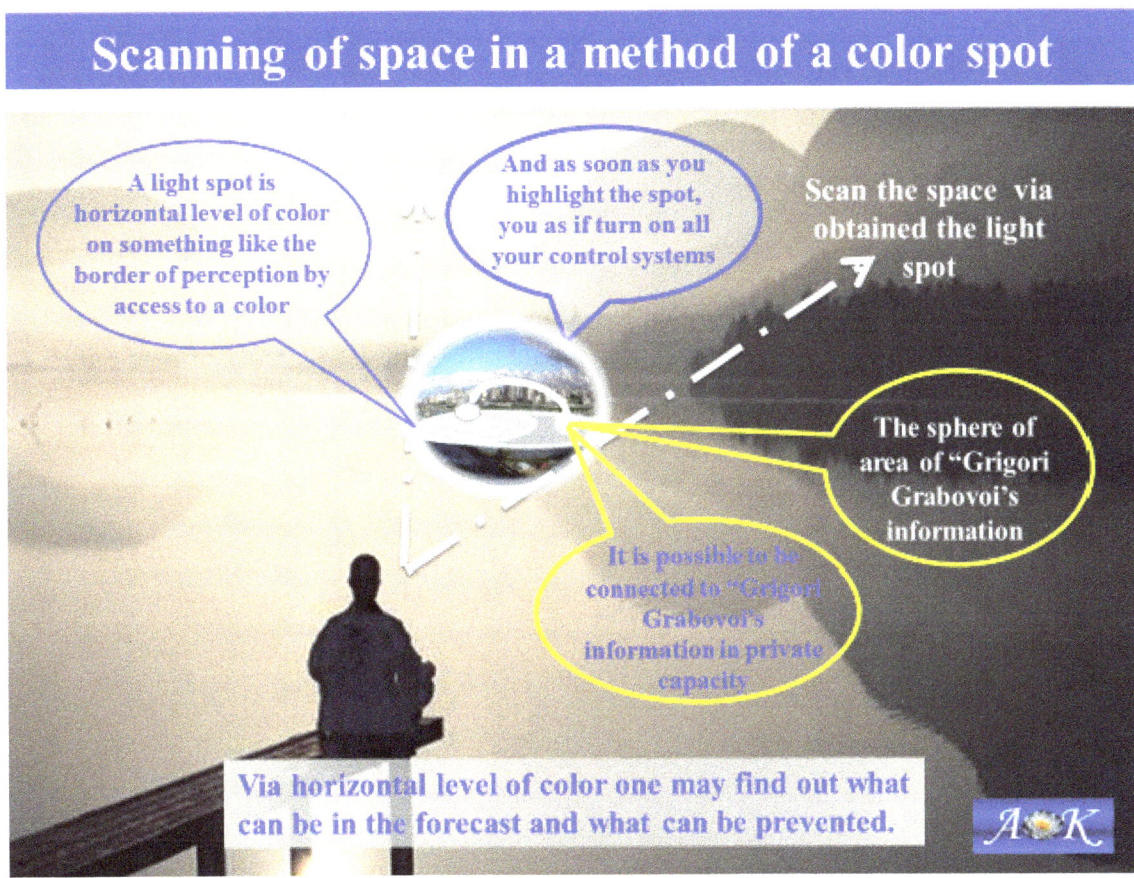

When cycle is over you can carry out scanning of space, of time. Via horizontal level of color one may find out what can be in the forecast and what can be prevented.

It is a quite good tool by the level of additional receipt of information from the area you have already detected. Scan information and take it behind the lens, the light spot. Obtained area is immediately perceived like a light spot and there is no need to work out in details, synchronize with known systems, for example. This color spot is just like a color plate, by the way, situated on something like the border of perception by access to a color somewhere near the body.

And as soon as you highlight the spot, you as if turn on all your control systems. Private procedure is as follows: you highlight a spot, divide it into two parts, make control – and you found the details in private capacity. If you highlight private tasks, you can connect directly to "Grigori Grabovoi's information". There is a nuance in case of highlighting of the other private tasks that is why it is desirable to consult with the original or to read the whole Author's text.

For example, Grigori Petrovich says that it is possible to distinguish a private number of tasks which is preserved after your first action and outlines the space around light spot. It turns out that it is necessary to find private tasks not in the space behind the light spot, but in the space of control which is highlighted by this color spot by connecting the sphere of "Grigori Grabovoi's information". In such cases you simply need practice.

If control must be continued after the first iteration with silver-white color, then start building color grades: you can color the left part with one color and the right part with the other color. Color selection is at your own discretion.

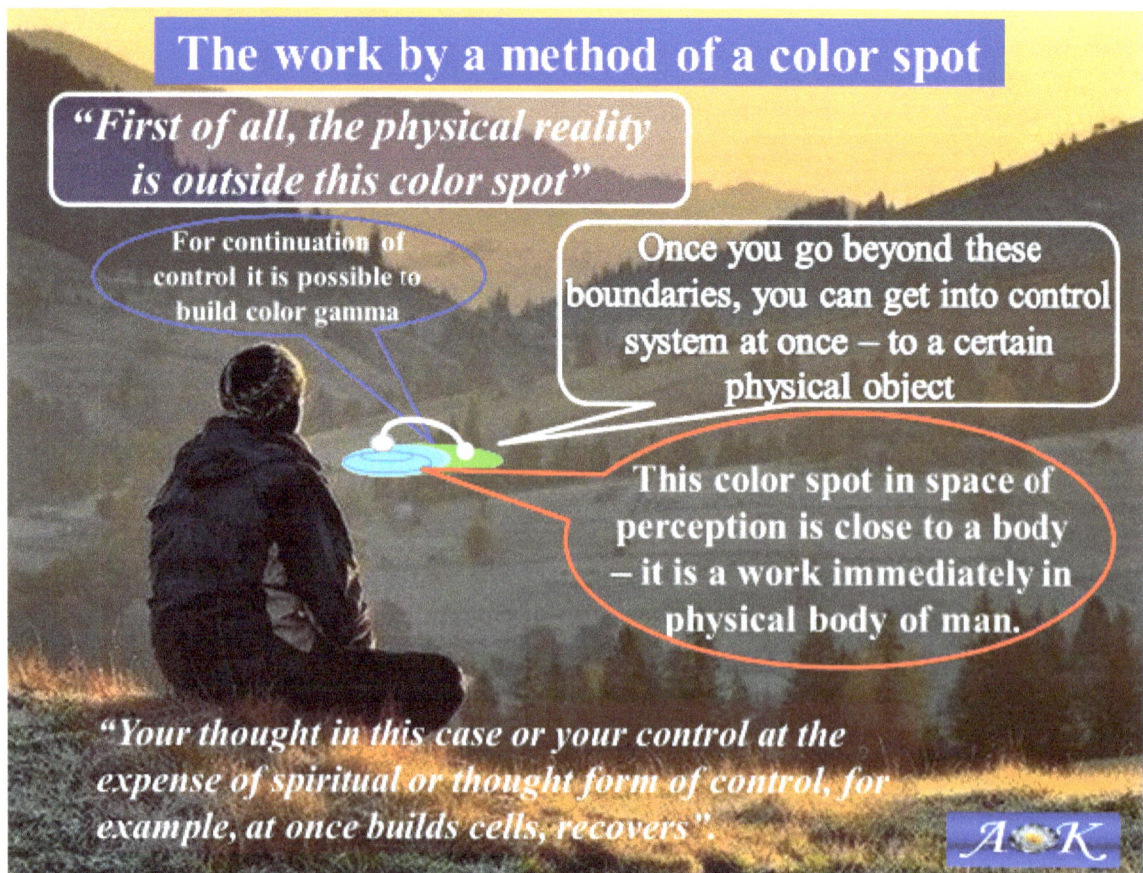

The work by a method of a color spot

"First of all, the physical reality is outside this color spot"

For continuation of control it is possible to build color gamma

Once you go beyond these boundaries, you can get into control system at once – to a certain physical object

This color spot in space of perception is close to a body – it is a work immediately in physical body of man.

"Your thought in this case or your control at the expense of spiritual or thought form of control, for example, at once builds cells, recovers".

An important level of reality in control is that *what* is located outside this color spot. *"First of all, the physical reality is outside this color spot".* It is even not a space of thinking, it is not the closest level where Spirit action exists. Once you go beyond these boundaries, you can get into control system at once – to a certain physical object.

If you approach this color spot to physical body of man in space of perception, you immediately work in physical body of man. *"And if then you control this process, you can see that your thought in this case or your control at the expense of spiritual or thought form of control, for example, at once builds cells, recovers".*

On the basis of technologies of these lectures it is necessary to have universal perception systems not only for distribution among everyone, but, the most important – they must be correctly described.

29. Control on color – separation of external part of control in respect of control goal

It is very simple control method. There is no need for you to think over that what will happen inside the system: you simply separate the whole external system in respect of control goal.

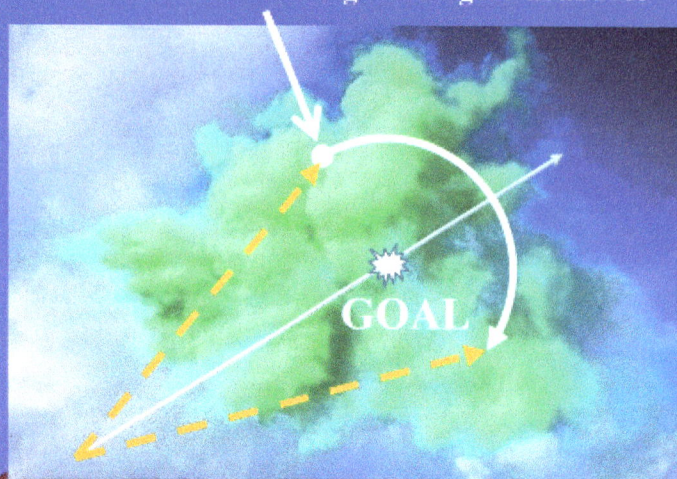

THE METHOD OF CONTROL ON COLOR IS GRIGORI GRABOVOI'S TECHNOLOGY

The area of the Teachings of Grigori Grabovoi

GOAL

There is no need for you to think over that what will happen inside the system: you simply separate the whole external system in respect of control goal.

It is very simple control method.

In external system we simply select the line or any element of color which corresponds to the area of the Teachings of Grigori Grabovoi on prevention of probable global catastrophe. This line is better to be introduced in white, silver-white color, for example.

It is advisable to move clockwise, that is, to move the hand with the area of the Teachings to the right from the level opposite of heart. Control area is a kind of spot of light but already fuzzy because there is no need to separate control details: the spot is in the center of selected external system.

Start moving clockwise – you can do it in less than no time – and immediately find a line which goes from this level in the center which is the goal of control. Fix any element of lighting which is the control system.

Control scheme:

- select in infinite space any element via which control takes place, that is, you are as a kind of control center;
- control is simple and very quick in this case, it is comparable

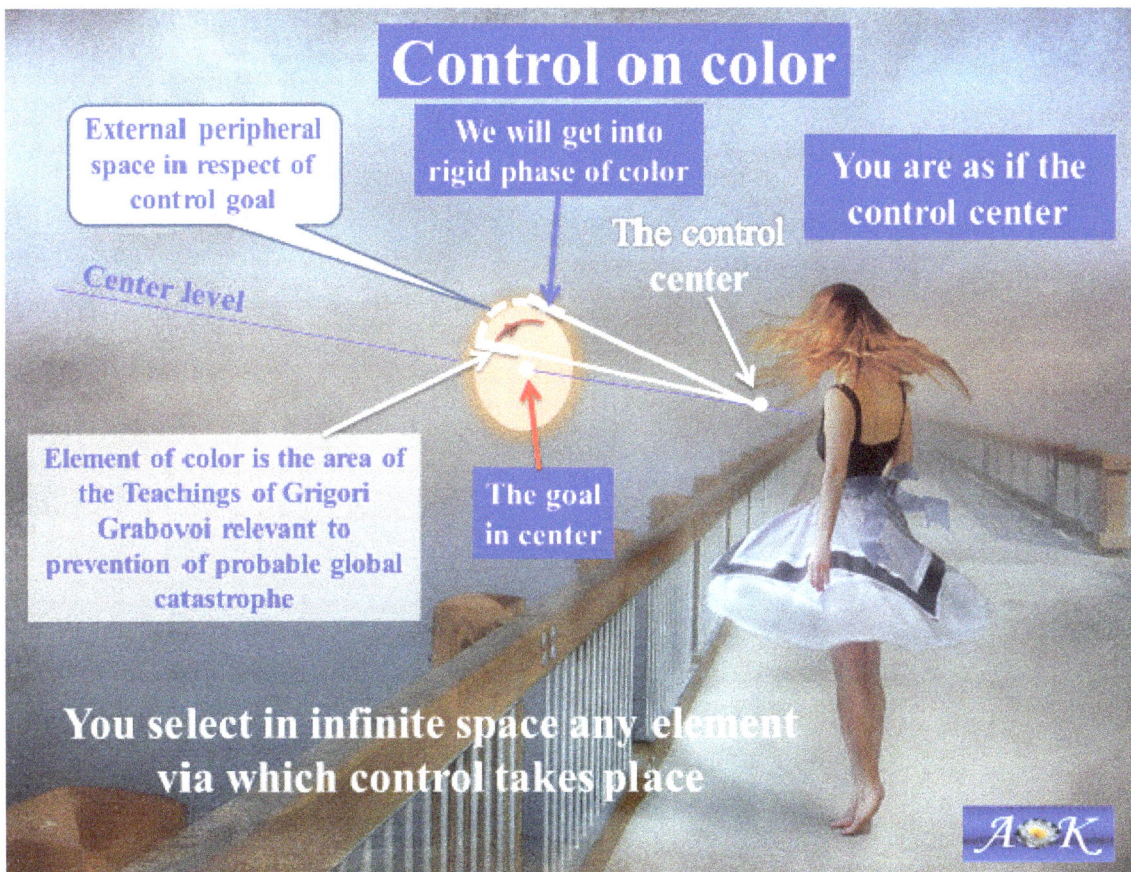

Control on color

External peripheral space in respect of control goal

We will get into rigid phase of color

You are as if the control center

The control center

Center level

Element of color is the area of the Teachings of Grigori Grabovoi relevant to prevention of probable global catastrophe

The goal in center

You select in infinite space any element via which control takes place

with the principle of instant control;

- selection of the central spot in control, in the central area without any special characteristics;
- it is enough to hold the goal at a spiritual level and select the central part of control;
- and also all external peripherical space is selected;
- in the left part – and it is better to be closer to heart – the area of the Teachings which corresponds to prevention of probable global catastrophe shall be selected. And moving almost immediately to the right – you can see it later – we will get into rigid phase of color;

- as soon as we fix this rigid phase of color, control takes place.

There are only three elements of action in this level of control:

  ➢ this is the selection of control area without going into the system;
  ➢ then selection of the color relevant to the area of the Teachings on prevention of probable global catastrophe;
  ➢ and the next action is clockwise in respect of you. This is the selection of control center.

It is necessary to repeat this method for several times: the more you repeat it, the faster you find direct control route where a conic control principle appears – and already volume one. It is possible to use not volume principle but movement clockwise from the right to the left in respect of physical body.

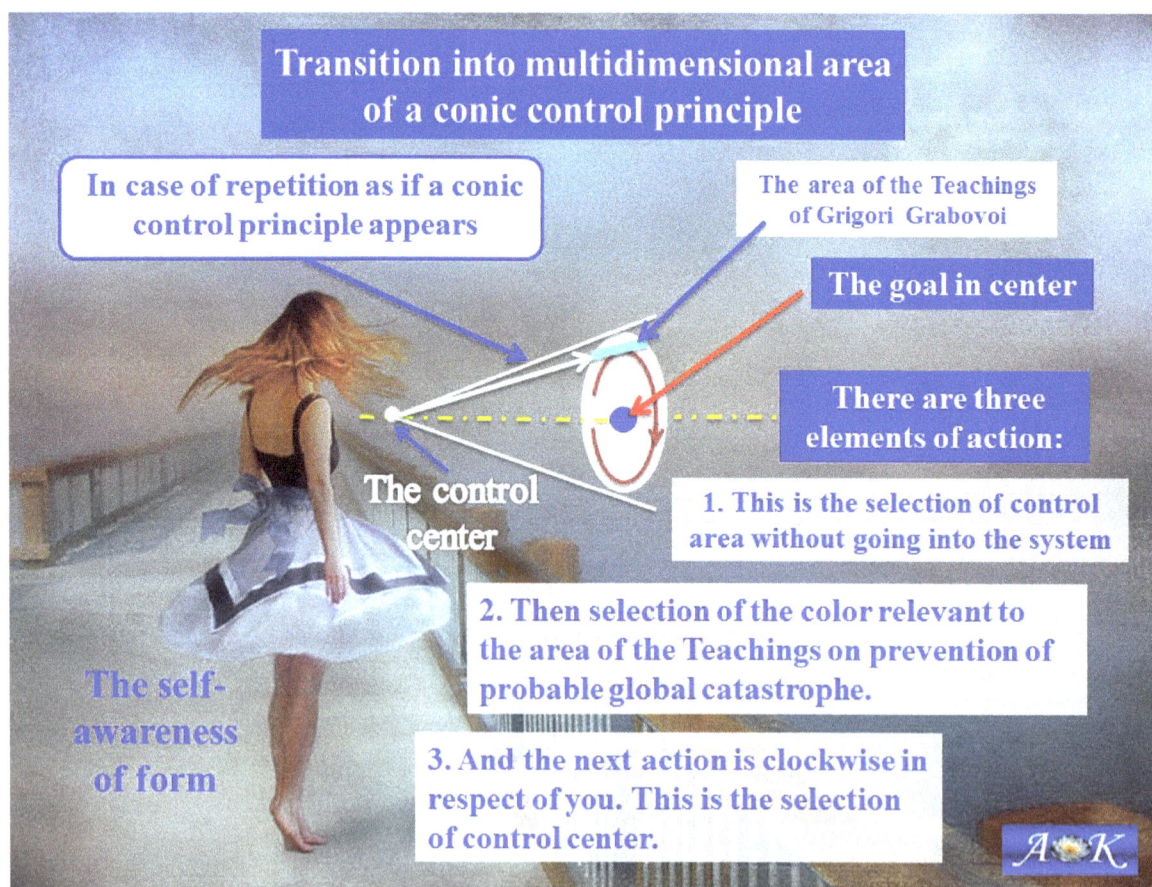

Transition into multidimensional area of a conic control principle

In case of repetition as if a conic control principle appears

The area of the Teachings of Grigori Grabovoi

The goal in center

There are three elements of action:

The control center

1. This is the selection of control area without going into the system

2. Then selection of the color relevant to the area of the Teachings on prevention of probable global catastrophe.

3. And the next action is clockwise in respect of you. This is the selection of control center.

The self-awareness of form

Transition into multidimensional area is the self-awareness of form: recognition of these principles gives control. *"It turns out that any task which comes to you can be solved".* The task is to fix only two things as clock hands: one line is the area of the Teachings of Grigori Grabovoi relevant to prevention of probable global catastrophe, *"and the second line is that what fixation is – it is that what you should pay attention to for control to take place and to take place immediately".*

And as far as you always know your own form, any questions with which people come to you in search for telepathy, you solve them based on your goals, even when you sleep and so on: it is rather autonomous system from the system of permanent concentration at the expense of Consciousness. Nevertheless, these control methods can be used at the usual time.

In case of collective concentration of Consciousness concerning certain questions, laws, if you make concentration in optical system, then access can be very bright: collective phase can be highlighted very quickly and strongly. You can determine even certain colors by concentrations – if we say that is it only silver-white or white color – anyway collective phase is manifested very quickly and dimensionally – percentage per a unit of Collective Consciousness will be high there.

In principle this system works even when man sleeps. Control takes place by some optical beam, that is, by color or light: many things will be very familiar and clear.

30. Method of control – color shred

The fifth method of color control covered by this course of lectures is as follows: you separate space around yourself, that is, around physical body in the form of light-enriched area – as if a searchlight lights. This searchlight does not light from anywhere, it is you who is the source of such vertical light pole.

Light level at the level of logical phase of representation is described in the seminar as follows: you stand in an infinite space – a very strong light illuminates starting from the level of your legs and it lights up, vectorially up. The light higher has a dense lighting in the area of shoulders and it loses vector direction. Vector of this lighting is from the level of feet to the area of shoulders, then background lighting happens.

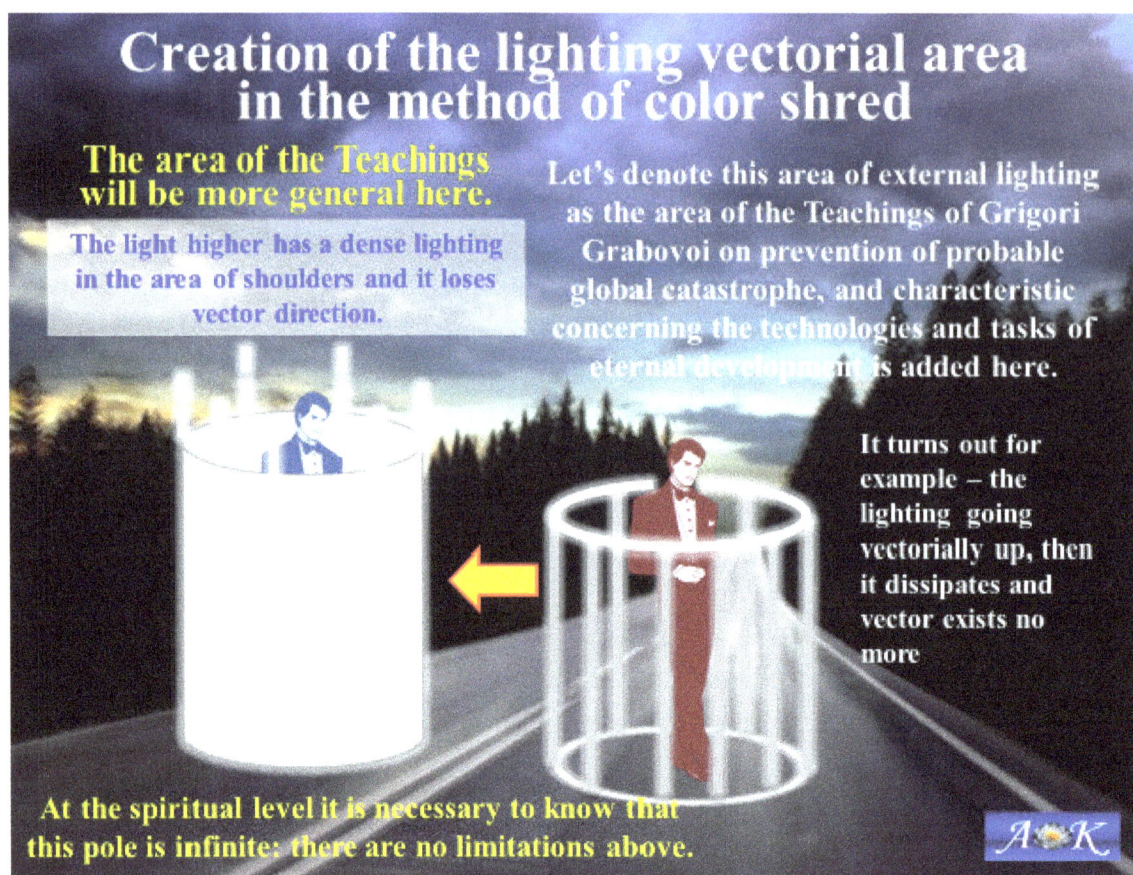

Creation of the lighting vectorial area in the method of color shred

The area of the Teachings will be more general here.

The light higher has a dense lighting in the area of shoulders and it loses vector direction.

Let's denote this area of external lighting as the area of the Teachings of Grigori Grabovoi on prevention of probable global catastrophe, and characteristic concerning the technologies and tasks of eternal development is added here.

It turns out for example – the lighting going vectorially up, then it dissipates and vector exists no more

At the spiritual level it is necessary to know that this pole is infinite: there are no limitations above.

Let's denote this area of external lighting as the area of the Teachings of Grigori Grabovoi on prevention of probable global catastrophe, and characteristic concerning the technologies and tasks of eternal development is added here. The area of the Teachings will be more general here.

And this external lighting can be manifested at once in any color more peculiar for you: and it is better to be closer to light color – better white with silver, but there can be light halftones at once. You can imagine lighting from only one side, it is not necessary to imagine this pole rigidly as a cylinder. Simply at the spiritual level it is necessary to know that this pole which wraps you is infinite: there are no limitations above.

The area of control goal in the form of colour shred is placed between your physical body and this light pole around you where its boundaries start: this can be 20-25 cm from body. It is better to place control goal in the form of color: let's think that recovery is a certain color. We place it opposite to the heart at the left.

Take a light shred of any color, which is called control goal. This is the work at the level of Soul that goes via the color: we do not work there with the systems manifested at the logical phase. So, take this kind of color shred and put above logical phase of control as with the will phase above the head – and give infinite characteristics concerning realization.

Take it above the head where color intensity is high – exactly of fundamental plan of the Creator –the lighting which has an infinite level of access in any phase starts there. And then take and quickly put it back where you formed the goal: take above and put back.

Method of color shred. The area of control goal and control scheme

Infinite characteristics concerning realization

Creator's level

You put control goal – color shred – with the will phase above the head

Creator's level

The lighting which has the infinite level of access in any phase starts

And then take and quickly put it back where you formed the goal.

The area of control goal in the form of color shred is placed between your physical body and this light pole around you where its boundaries start: this can be 20-25 cm from body.
Place it opposite to the heart.

Here realization takes place as far as quick access to infinite area happens: while we are dragging this color piece it can as if become smaller. While we are dragging one volume – the goal is already realized, then take color up – it is something like a photon – it starts flying apart.

"Then place it back – it can be not exactly the same, but you simply know that even one point of such color contains your goal – a kind of shred which can already have no clear boundaries at the edges: instead of rectangle a circle or similar shape can appear. Put it back and fix. Well, you are free not to place it back, if you want you can take it only above".

Repetition of control scheme:

- ➢ lighting which goes vectorially up and is designated by the area of the Teachings starts;
- ➢ then it dissipates and vector exists no more;
- ➢ the goal in respect to your body, for example, is a very small shred of color – you must see the place of this shred in respect of this light pole and in respect of you;
- ➢ for quick and precise realization of control goal it is important to fix the coordinate: you internally evaluate the location, as if look at the internal plan where the shred is located and remember this place;
- ➢ then you can simply move up – you bring to the level of control according to the law of the Creator, to the law of eternal life – and that is all;
- ➢ you can also take it back to the same place.

Method of color shred. The area of control goal

The lighting which has the infinite level of access in any phase begins

Let's denote this area of external lighting as the area of the Teachings of Grigori Grabovoi on prevention of probable global catastrophe, and characteristic concerning the technologies and tasks of eternal development is added here.

The shred of color – the goal of control is placed opposite to the heart between a body and an area of a light, then put above the head.

You receive control but without the level of consecutive characteristics: control is carried out in such a way as if there was no influence. *"For example, it can be so that a piece of tissue, organ simply grows up as if it was always there, but if it wasn't there and so on, or the event took place, but it is so harmonious, that in principle the world develops exactly in such a way – it is something like according to the laws of development of the world, universe".*

And the spiritual vision of own usual physical form is essential here, because in this case you control over your form too – the form which is restructured in the perception into light. When consequential part takes place you work in the phase where the Spirit organizes the body. *"And this is the principle of eternal control, eternal development of body – by its own".*

"And when you use this level, you can make, generally speaking, any control also because structure of eternity is an infinite control, and if it is with an infinite access of light, then it turns out that you can realize any event always in case of preciseness of coordinate system".

Accuracy of understanding of technologies is very important, it is often given in the Author's text, in transitions, explanations, sometimes in repetitions, comparisons and so on. That is why first of all it is important to listen to or watch the seminar itself, when you have face-to-face communication with Grabovoi Grigori Petrovich.

An special control for increase of speed characteristics of some color in relation to white

The level of control according to the law of the Creator, to the law of eternal life

The goal is increase of speed characteristics of selected color

Lighting is the area of the Teachings of Grigori Grabovoi on prevention of probable global catastrophe plus structure of eternity

Scheme of control:
• lighting which goes vectorially up starts;
• then it dissipates and vector exists no more;
• you must see the place of this shred in respect of this light pole and in respect of you;
• it is important to fix the coordinate: you internally evaluate the location, where the shred is located and remember this place;
• then you can simply move up the goal;
• you can also take the goal back to the same place.

"When you work with any color, you should adhere to such a rule, if possible: any other color, except white and silver white, should not decrease control speed in your perception if it is possible".

In some cases you should intentionally increase, if necessary, control constructions of speed of control distribution, if you work with color. For example, you think that it is this color which can work in this situation, then you intentionally make control for increase of speed characteristics of color. Such situation happens that you as if refresh color. *"It is possible to create vivid independent systems that constantly realise the goal of your control even if you set it once, because they are simply synchronized with the systems from the life in color".*

FIVE CONTROL METHODS BY MEANS OF SOUNDS AND FORMS
THREE METHODS COVER CONTROL BY MEANS OF SOUNDS.

31. Control through the level of general sound

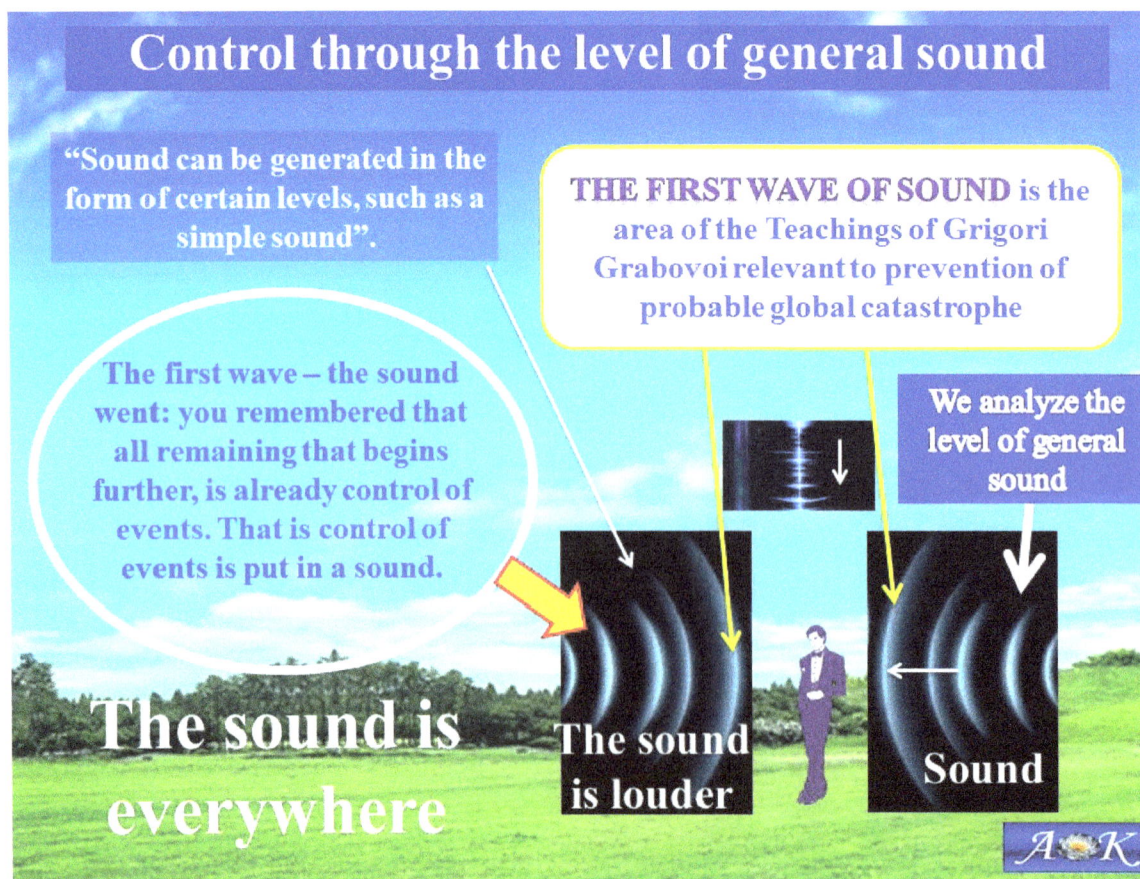

Control through the level of general sound

"Sound can be generated in the form of certain levels, such as a simple sound".

THE FIRST WAVE OF SOUND is the area of the Teachings of Grigori Grabovoi relevant to prevention of probable global catastrophe

The first wave – the sound went: you remembered that all remaining that begins further, is already control of events. That is control of events is put in a sound.

We analyze the level of general sound

The sound is everywhere

The sound is louder

Sound

Educational course of control ends up with rather easy material. The first control method by means of sound lies in the fact that you analyze the level of general sound which is around you. And there are no limitations, no forms – there is just sound there.

After analyzing the level of general sound we designate the first wave of sound as the area of the Teachings of Grigori Grabovoi relevant to section of prevention of probable global catastrophe. It is necessary to separate clearly that the first what we hear after starting to generate sound is the area of the Teachings. *"Sound can be generated in the form of certain levels, such as a simple sound".*

Control scheme:
  ❖ analyze the level of general sound;
  ❖ correlate the first wave of sound with the area of the Teachings of Grigori Grabovoi relevant to prevention of probable global catastrophe;
  ❖ remember what is further – the sound which has control for your task, for example, control over the event.

32. Control through local sound wave

The second method lies in the fact that during control the wave approaching to us is perceived as the sound. *"It is already a local system".* In the first method sound sounded everywhere around you, in this method sound goes from somewhere as a local wave: for example, the plane flies – the sound is heard locally, it is heard from one place – and you perceive approaching sound.

Designate the first wave of sound with the area of the Teachings of Grigori Grabovoi in part of prevention of probable global catastrophe and provision of eternal development. There are two components here: the area also possessed the level of provision of eternal development. As soon as we hear the first wave – it is the area of the Teachings by two components.

Further sound which you attract to you just like to a magnet is the control over your event. Sound may be different: you can separate a melody, you may separate simply a generation of erratic sound, like a roar of waves or breaking of waves. In this method the sound is selected individually – it can be a dog's barking – no problem if you think that dog's barking controls.

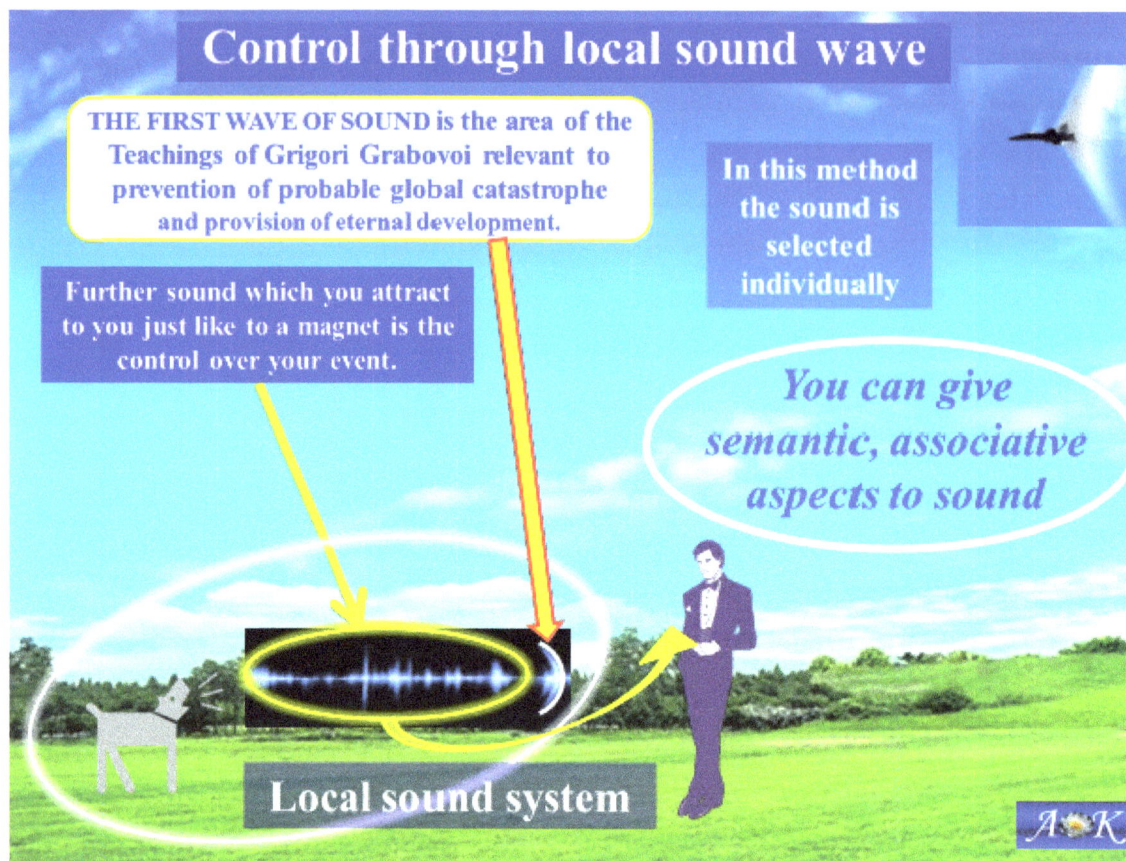

By the way, it is really so that if dog barks it blocks the way to somebody, and it is already a control system. *"That is, you can give semantic, associative aspects to sound".*

33. Generation of sound near oneself

The third control method by means of sound *"lies in the fact that you start generating sound around you and push it from yourself with a wave".* The first wave of generation – which you generate – this wave corresponds to the area of the Teachings of Grigori Grabovoi in the part of prevention of probable global catastrophe. Here this part is reviewed alone. The next what you generate is actually a control goal.

There is one general principle in these three methods – you formulate control goal, *"that is, you set control goal at the level of thinking, and then you make these actions with sound putting control for goal realization into the sound".* For example, a general sound system works, then the principle is as follows: the more such sound you generate the more control you make.

Generation of sound near oneself

"You set control goal at the level of thinking, and then you make these actions with sound putting control for goal realization into the sound".

The first wave of a generating sound is the wave relevant to the area of the Teachings of Grigori Grabovoi in the part of prevention of probable global catastrophe.

For example, a general sound system works, then the principle is as follows: the more such sound you generate the more control you make.

"You as if work with endless level", then your control immediately becomes general.

At the moment of generation you can see light forms: for example, the wave – it is visible because you anyway see, just like a silvery outline of a chaotic wave or like a patch of sunlight. *"You can see it or you cannot see it, you can work simply with sound, but you can as if see how the wave looks like... For example, it is better for a musician to work with a sound but without light-optical images: that is why he clearly understands what the wave at a spiritual level is, but he can fail to perceive light optics".*

During realization of infinite development of sound wave – generation of sound around yourself – you have no limitations.

Property of sound is used here – any sound fragmentation, as far as there is no limitations here, for example, in space and time, then in this case sound is like an absolute system which propagates exactly in the space of perception. *"And that is why it turns out that you as if work with infinite level, you do not restrict yourself to carrying platform for control":* then your control immediately becomes general.

The principle of generality means that you work exactly with the notion of sound – you do not work even with light optics which exist, but can be non-concentrated, for example. And sound is the main characteristic of this work.

CONTROL BY MEANS OF FORMS

34. Control through silver-white sphere

The first method of control by means of forms is very easy. The method lies in the fact that you introduce into control a sphere which is located at any place. The form of sphere is silver-white in color and it is imagined or perceived at any place, that is, its location is not fixed anywhere.

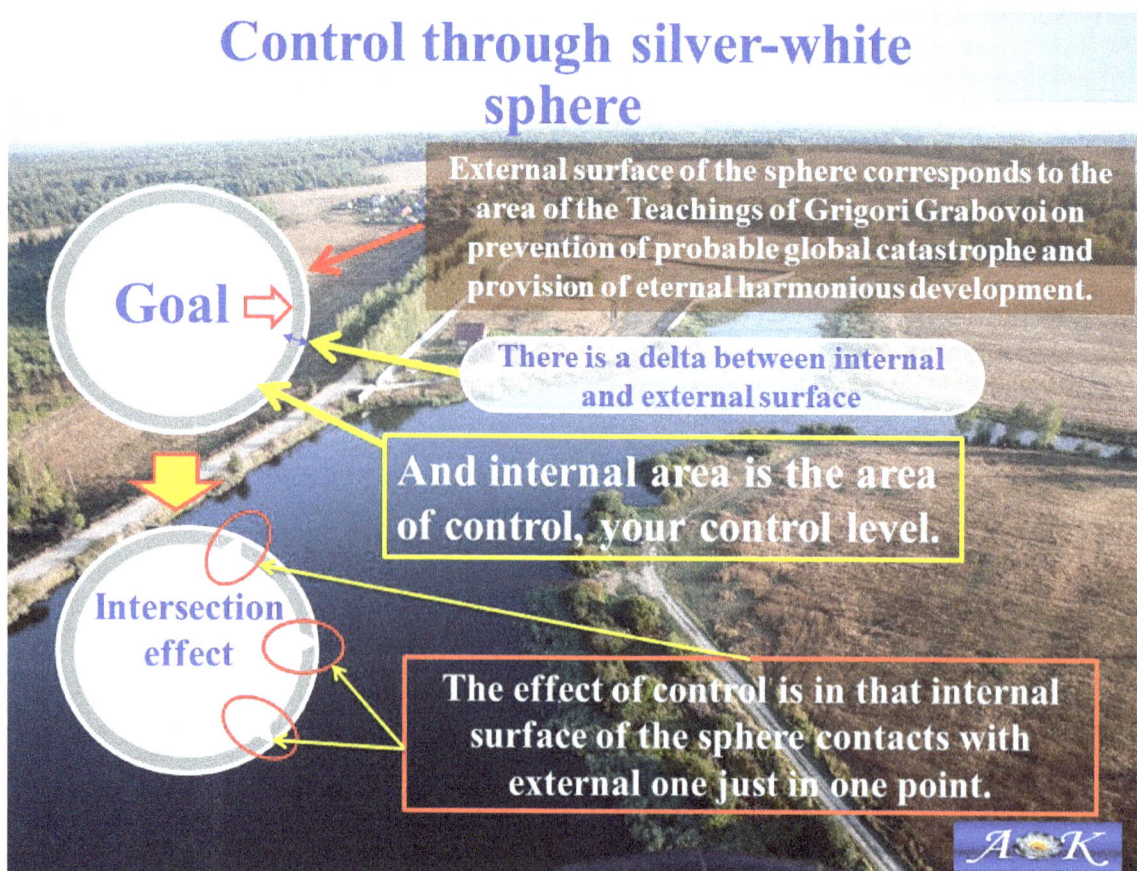

Control through silver-white sphere

Goal ⇨

External surface of the sphere corresponds to the area of the Teachings of Grigori Grabovoi on prevention of probable global catastrophe and provision of eternal harmonious development.

There is a delta between internal and external surface

And internal area is the area of control, your control level.

Intersection effect

The effect of control is in that internal surface of the sphere contacts with external one just in one point.

In this sphere external surface corresponds to the area of the Teachings of Grigori Grabovoi on prevention of probable global catastrophe and provision of eternal harmonious development. And internal area is the area of control, your control level. And the task - the first control element - is to divide these two levels.

"As far as external surface is familiar, you fix internal surface of sphere in your Consciousness". There is a delta between internal and external surface. You often work with internal surface: hold the control goal in Consciousness.

Here we have an effect of accessibility of control. The effect of control is in that internal surface of the sphere contacts with external one just in one point. Intersection effect as a rule lights up in the form of one point at such background level of lighting. *"And you receive control effect, that is, you performed control cycle".* In principle, you can create more points, that is, fix at many points on surface. And further – you have no problems.

35. Transition of flat form of triangle into the volume of infinite pole

Control by means of form in the second method lies in the fact that at first you separate a triangle in space of perception which is transformed into a conic form with the foundation downward, then the form of cone is introduced into infinite vertical pole.

And this vertical pole is the area of the Teachings of Grigori Grabovoi relevant to prevention of probable global catastrophe and provision of eternal harmonious development. Initial control level: the pole starts highlighting the cone. *"The cone itself highlighted in this pole is the control goal: I mean such a simple cone".*

This control method by means of form is a principle of transition of finite form into eternal one. *"And the effect of control lies in the transition. That is, the effect of control lies not even in the form. The peculiarity of spiritual control lies here. It is the same as the transition of a logical phase into the Spirit: and we receive control effect at the expense of transfer of finite form into infinite one".*

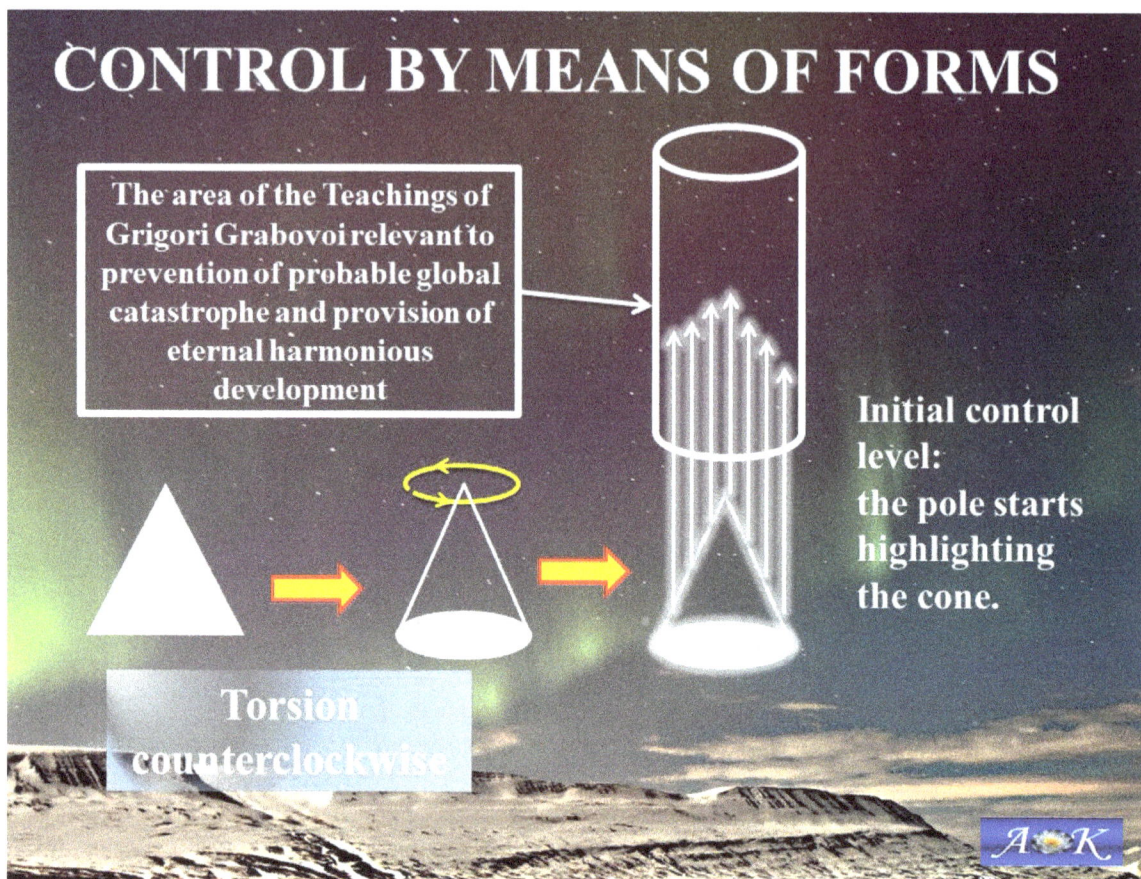

Control scheme in this method is as follows:
1. first of all we have a triangle in the area of perception;
2. a cone is generated by means of moving the triangle counter clockwise. You can simply perceive cone immediately;
3. the cone transits – the lighting as if starts going up;
4. the lighting going up as if breaks downward – an infinite vertical pole appears.

The external lighting is an infinite cylinder. Cylindrical surface is the area of the Teachings of Grigori Grabovoi relevant to prevention of probable global catastrophe and provision of eternal harmonious development. Control area is a cone surface which is highlighted with silver-white light of this control pole.

"Control is such that we receive dimensional and then infinite form from finite and rather simple and flat form. And the infinite form itself acts in a highlighted part as a control aspect of the goal".

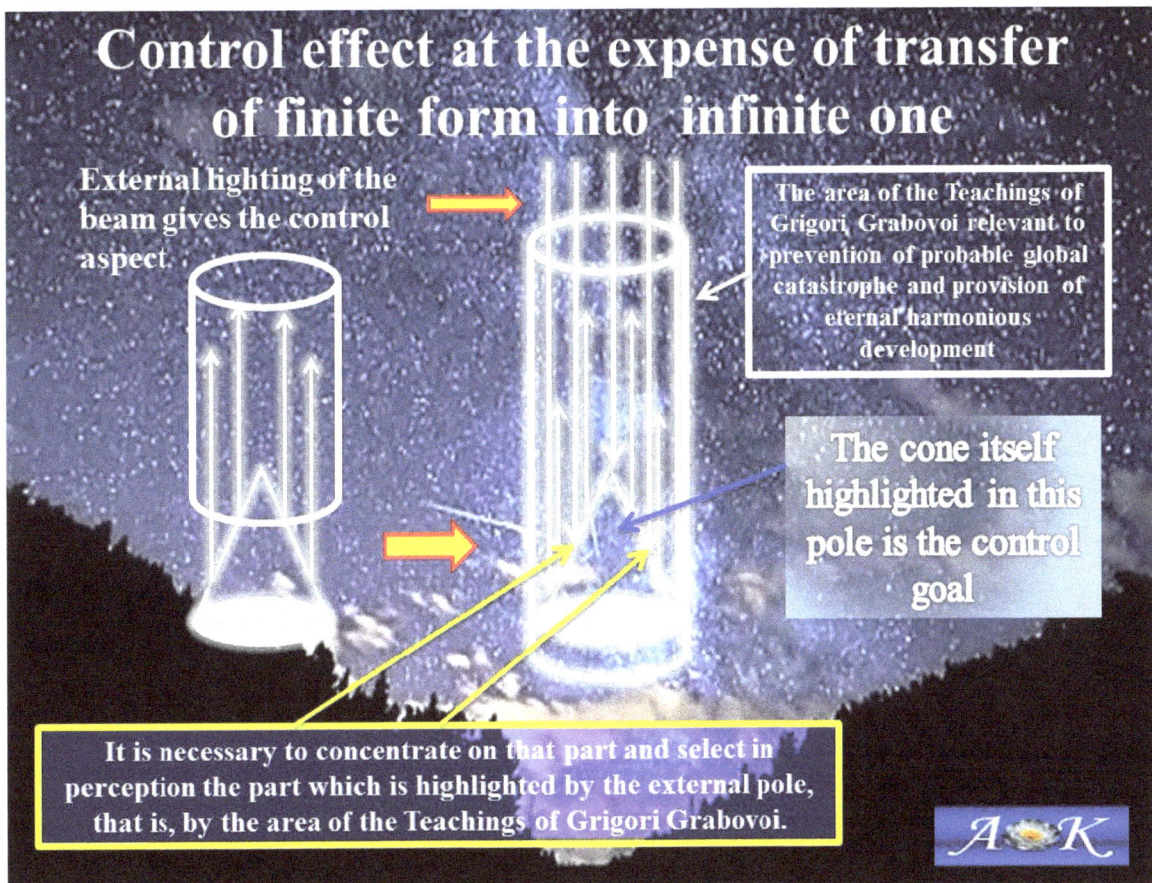

At first the beam lights from the cone. Simple logical development shows that return lighting of the beam from above – external lighting – gives the control aspect. Light can be more manifested on the cone, somewhere in different way. It is necessary to concentrate on that part and select in perception the part which is highlighted by the external pole, that is, by the area of the Teachings of Grigori Grabovoi.

Five methods are absolutely simple and they use such known notions as sound and form. Nothing else is used here. In the second method of control by form the notion of infinite pole is used, but it is that what can be studied later: it is generally recommended to study the details of this control.

Grabovoi G.P.: "Here you can see that when, for example, we make general control, then in fact we make the general development more intensive, that is, we immediately transfer knowledge to everyone – the next knowledge which you mastered at the expense of your technologies, at the expense of the fact that you taught somebody, at the expense of the fact that you solved your tasks. And other people mastered and also solved their tasks and transfer their knowledge to others. And it turns out that it is the other light – it is the light created by people, where people can make general control and they can independently solve personal tasks and the tasks of everyone, of the whole civilization and, of course, the tasks of eternal development. Surely, in any case the God will always help people". (The Teachings of Grigori Grabovoi about God. General influence of God, June 16, 2004).

List of references:

1. Grabovoi G.P., **"Lecture 1. Introduction** – for lecturers of initial training", April 16, 2002;

2. Grabovoi G.P., **"LIT. Lecture 2.** System of salvation and harmonious development of Grigori Grabovoi. Methods of control by means of concentration on numbers or creation of number series", April 23, 2002;

3. Grabovoi G.P., **"LIT. Lecture 3.** System of salvation and harmonious development. Control by means of phrases. Eight methods", May 14, 2002;

4. Grabovoi G.P., **"LIT. Lecture 4.** System of salvation and harmonious development. Technology and methods of control by means of color", May 22, 2002;

5. Grabovoi G.P., **"LIT. Lecture 5.** Technology of salvation and harmonious development. Methods of control by means of sound and forms", May 27, 2002;

6. Grabovoi G.P., "The methods of promotion of Grigori Grabovoi's works in social networks", 2006;

7. Grabovoi G.P., "The Teachings of Grigori Grabovoi about God. General influence of God", June 16, 2004.

www.ingramcontent.com/pod-product-compliance
Lightning Source LLC
Chambersburg PA
CBHW042055220326

41599CB00042BA/7220